DYNAMICS OF
HEALTH CARE

DYNAMICS OF HEALTH CARE

Third Edition

Ruth M. French, M.A.
Associate Dean
School of Associated Medical Sciences
College of Medicine
University of Illinois at the Medical Center

McGraw-Hill Book Company

New York   St. Louis   San Francisco   Auckland   Bogotá   Düsseldorf
Johannesburg   London   Madrid   Mexico   Montreal   New Delhi
Panama   Paris   São Paulo   Singapore   Sydney   Tokyo   Toronto

DYNAMICS OF HEALTH CARE

2 3 4 5 6 7 8 9 0   MUMU   7 8 3 2 1 0 9

This book was set in Times Roman by The Total Book (ECU/BTI).
The editor was Stuart D. Boynton; the production
supervisor was Jeanne Selzam.
The Murray Printing Company was printer and binder.

CONTENTS

PREFACE

He who knows nothing, loves nothing. He who can do nothing understands nothing. He who understands nothing is worthless. But he who understands, also loves, notices, sees. The more knowledge is inherent in a thing, the greater the love. Anyone who imagines that all fruits ripen at the same time as strawberries knows nothing about grapes.

Paracelsus

Paracelsus has stated the case for this book and the basis for my writing it for those of us in the health care field. There is a real need for knowing more about the context within which we work—the people and the institutions—before we can understand, appreciate, and seek opportunities for the creative cooperation that is so essential in this age of specialization.

Suggestions for improvements and additional topics to be covered have been carefully weighed, and some of them are incorporated in this edition. Others were omitted for reasons relating to the problems posed by the rapid changes in the economic, social, and legislative climates, as well as in the health care field itself. For example, one has to decide whether to include data that may soon be obsolete, or alternatively to risk the criticism of superficiality by merely alluding to such data and referring the reader to sources from which current data may be obtained. Another problem is posed by the proliferation of health-related work groups (through the fragmentation of existing professions or because of new needs) whose professional status may be just emerging or else doubtful. Obviously, the chapter on health services personnel does not cover all health-related work groups.

The beginnings of systematic efforts to breach the barriers that separate health personnel with regard to both function and professional education are encouraging. However, there is a long way to go before the goal of genuine teamwork is reached. In writing this book, I hope to make a contribution to efforts leading to the achievement of that goal.

The list of persons who offered help, interest, and encouragement in the writing of this book is too long to make it possible to identify individuals. Nevertheless, I would like to express my appreciation to all those persons, and especially to the students and colleagues with whom I worked at St. Louis University and the University of Illinois at the Medical Center. Evidence of that appreciation can best be seen in my efforts to achieve a high level of quality in both writing and content.

Ruth M. French

INTRODUCTION

A common suggestion for this edition of *Dynamics of Health Care* was to include more references to more of the health-related fields among the examples used. Recognizing that the chances of pleasing everyone in every instance are slim, and believing that teachers can best add their own flavors to instruction by use of examples that are both topical and specific to given professions, I have not attempted to cover every field in the examples cited.

Teachers should be able to use a textbook as a springboard as well as a source of information, and thus facilitate their students in thinking for themselves. The skeleton, or framework, of information and ideas presented in the text can be fleshed out and molded to suit the needs of students and teachers alike. My approach has been with this in mind, in the expectation that the physical therapists, for example, will add special knowledge and experience in terms of the physical therapist's role to make what I have written come alive to students. Role modeling can be an important part of the educational process in this manner.

I have elected not to include study questions at the conclusion of each chapter for two reasons: first, the teacher's function is to identify objectives for the students' learning, and since I could not presume to know what they might be, I could not pose questions that would be related to those objectives. Secondly, I find that most such study questions tend to be at the recall level, testing for facts rather than for interpretation and problem solving that involve the higher cognitive taxonomic levels. My concern is that students use the information in their own thought processes rather than memorize it in bits and pieces.

DYNAMICS OF
HEALTH CARE

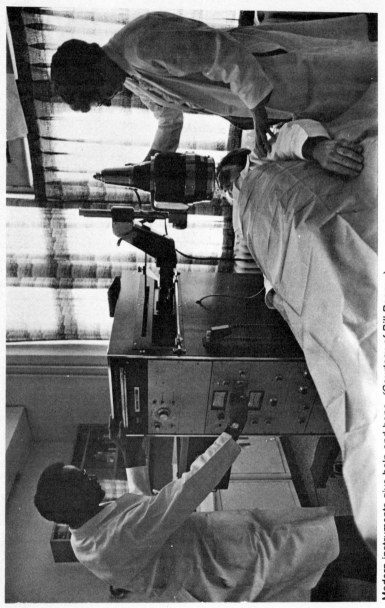

Modern instruments give help and hope. (*Courtesy of Bill Rogers.*)

1

OUR CONCERN: HEALTH

WHAT IS HEALTH?

The most comprehensive definition of health is stated in the charter of the World Health Organization (WHO): "the state of complete physical, mental, and social well-being and not merely the absence of disease or infirmity." If this concept of health is to be a guide, there is a need to extend the scope of involvement in health care planning and delivery. Although the principal efforts have been toward only the first part of the WHO definition of health, there are indications that more consideration is being given to mental and social well-being.

For example, both mental and social aspects are involved in the federal and local regulations and industrial codes governing programs that portray violence on television. The impetus for these regulations has come from various groups, predominately parents and teachers. These regulations have resulted in some reduction of the incidence and specificity of the depiction of violence. To many, the results have not been as satisfactory as desired, and the pressure is being continued to reduce the portrayal of violence still further.

The rise in pornography has generated strong reactions leading to legal action against purveyors of pornography, and local ordinances directed toward controlling the location and numbers of so-called adult bookshops and theaters featuring pornographic films. The principal issues at stake in these suits and regulations are those of definitions of violence and pornography, and the implied, if not actual, censorship that abridges the right of free speech.

Federal agencies have been established that have missions related to mental and social well-being. The Environmental Protection Agency is primarily concerned with health hazards, but also with the broader aspects of the quality of life. The Department of State has a Bureau of Population and Humanitarian Assistance, as well as an Office of Food for Peace. The Department of Health Education and Welfare (DHEW) has a Social and Rehabilitation Service, and the Department of Housing and Urban Development (HUD) has an Office for Environmental Quality.

Despite these developments, the natural tendency is to take a simplistic approach to the problems involved in health care, assuming that money and energy spent in prodigious amounts on medical research and service will alleviate these problems. We feel a need to limit our thinking to those areas in which we have some experience, reflecting Schopenhauer's observation[13] that "Every man takes the limits of his own field of vision as the limits of the world." But, as implied in the WHO definition of health, there is much more involved to which health practitioners must address themselves, and, in so doing, enlist the aid of experts in fields other than medicine. We have to face the fact that medical care is but one of the many elements contributing to health, even though an improvement in health is seen as a product of medically oriented effort. Success in dealing with problems of health is evaluated largely by such criteria of medical science as disease incidence and life expectancy. Even less precise, and more difficult to measure, are the profound influences of individual living habits, socioeconomic status, attitudes, housing, and education—the whole constellation of cultural and economic factors—on the degree of health enjoyed by our people.

There is a growing acceptance of the principle of homeostasis as a realistic and comprehensive overview in matters of health. This principle is implicit in the WHO definition. Simply stated, *homeostasis* is the maintenance of balance of conditions within a system. The term originated in physiology as a concept of one body with many functions, all of which are interdependent.[14]

The concept of homeostasis has been expanded beyond this relatively narrow application to include not only physiologic but mental and social aspects as well. One can think of it as the maintenance of (1) body balance, sometimes within very fine ranges; (2) psychologic and emotional balances; (3) cultural, social, and political balances; and (4) spiritual and philosophic balance. With this larger definition and application, health care can be a tremendous task, requiring efforts directed toward maintaining and, when needed, restoring balances within the individual and within his environment.

Disease or trauma is a threat to homeostasis, a threat which calls into action the protective and restorative mechanisms of the body. When the stress imposed is too great for the body to meet, medical or surgical intervention becomes necessary. The psychologic emotional, social, cultural, and spiritual balances must also be maintained, and these are subject—as are the physiologic—to checks, controls, and environmental adjustments. All relate to the physiologic homeostatic state and contribute to the ultimate behavior of the individual. Thus, all require the understanding of health services personnel, since they form the framework within which comprehensive health care is delivered.

Selye[14] conceptualizes disease as a result of stress which the body is incapable of overcoming. Exposure to stress causes both damage (shock) and defense (countershock). Disease, as old as life itself, *is* life. It is a manifestation of life through the reactions of a total living organism to abnormal stimuli. Disease is a consequence of interactions between organisms and environmental stimuli (which may be chemical, physical, biologic, sociologic, etc.), stimuli which exceed the adaptability of the subject. Subsequent reactions are no longer physiological, but pathophysiological, with limitation and impairment of further adaptability (freedom) of the organism.

These pathophysiological reactions are manifested by the signs and symptoms of disease.

IMPLICATIONS OF HEALTH

Throughout the world the wealth of nations is predicated upon the health of its people. Obviously, material resources, productivity, and consumption of goods and services are without meaning if the health of the people is such that it prevents their maximal utilization and activity. Economic prosperity is intimately associated with health. Hence, it is reasonable that programs of assistance to the developing nations of the world should include health care as one of their major points. To be sure, caring for the health of peoples is, in large measure, humanitarian, but its economic influence should not be overlooked. For example, Peace Corps members have been trained not only to teach such fundamentals as reading, or improving crop productivity, but also to participate in health-related activities appropriate to the areas in which they serve.

INFLUENCES ON MODERN HEALTH CARE

Attitudes as Determinants of Health Care

Interwoven among the strands making up the health of a people are the culturally related attitudes toward health itself, and toward the means of promoting health. The daily barrage of advertising and health articles in popular magazines suggests that ours is a culture bent on having the most healthy people on earth. However, the prevailing attitude seems to be that principles of good health are meant for the other fellow: "It can't happen to me." Directors of programs for early cancer detection have a difficult time persuading people to take advantage of the facilities provided for their benefit. This program, like many others, is resisted by those with an inherent fear of discovery of disease, who irrationally block out the obvious fact that treatment can be most successful at early stages, before symptoms have become manifest. Most Americans seem to have an attitude of utter faith, blithely believing that the status quo will never change. A telling example of the reactions of the general public to well-substantiated safety recommendations is shown by a study made by the National Safety Council. The president, Howard Pyle,[12] discussed drivers' attitudes toward seat belts and their use, citing the fact that, in 1964, only one out of twenty motorists had seat belts. Pyle makes the point that "while you can legislate seat belts into cars, you can't as easily legislate them around the waists of passengers." The study revealed that there was general agreement that seat belts save lives. But, paradoxically, seat belts remind people of accidents and invest them with a negative quality. The initial response to the study seemed to be that a seat-belt user is some kind of nut or sissy or an old fuddy-duddy. The task of selling the belts—and their use—to motorists has become easier by shifting the emphasis from disaster to success. One safety campaign device is a poster showing a racing driver fastening a seat belt; it is captioned "Professional advice about winning."

But even these campaigns and the reinforcements such as insurance company stipulations limiting coverage of injury if seat belts were not fastened at the time of an accident, and the use of a buzzer system that is turned off only when the seat belts are extended have not been universally heeded. Many people deactivate the seat-belt buzzer system. In apparent recognition of this habit, car manufacturers have changed the buzzer system so that it automatically turns off within a short time whether the seat belts are fastened or not.

Gaps between Knowledge and Acceptance

The attitude of the general public toward seat belts is as casual as its attitude toward cigarette smoking. The case against cigarette smoking is well documented and well publicized, yet, after a momentary drop in smoking following the announcement of medical findings, there was an increase in smoking. In part, the increase in smoking may be due to an increase in the numbers of persons at the "smoking permitted" level in our population. The figures suggest that new smokers, the former nonsmokers, are not intimidated by statistics. However, the nonsmokers have had significant influence on where smoking is permitted. Witness the separation of smoking and nonsmoking sections in aircraft and the increasing numbers of public gathering places such as restaurants and lounges that identify separate areas or prohibit smoking. Some states have laws prohibiting smoking in public places.

Involved in an odd collusion, the public is party to the reluctance of legislators to deal effectively with the tobacco industry by setting up controls similar to those governing other hazardous products. The Food and Drug Administration bans products that are implicated as carcinogens, yet all the Public Health Service can do is require that a warning be printed on cigarette packages. DHEW Secretary Joseph Califano has instituted a campaign to reduce smoking, depending on educational approaches. On being asked about the discrepancy between government action in campaigning against smoking while at the same time providing subsidies to tobacco growers, Secretary Califano responded that "Tobacco subsidies don't make people want to smoke. If they did, I would seek changes." This response does not seem logical, however. The dilemma is one of economics—the tobacco industry, including growers, is big business, viewed from any perspective.

A wide gap obviously separates scientific knowledge and public acceptance of that knowledge. The public may ignore valuable information or make indiscriminate use of it. To be sure, there must be a proper balance between overenthusiastic, indiscriminate application and outright rejection of both ideas and products. Too often a new drug or procedure is hailed as the answer to myriad problems, only to be discredited later because it cannot live up to the unrealistically high expectations; then, as experience and wisdom are gained, proper regard is finally reached.

Consider the response to the discovery of antibiotics. These potent drugs have been used to treat a wide range of infections, some of which are amenable to other modes of treatment, and the result has been the creation of more serious problems such as the development of strains of organisms that are resistant to antibiotics; the individual's development of an allergy to the drug, thus precluding its use when it could be the treatment of choice; or suppression by the antibiotic of bone marrow hematopoeisis, with life-threatening results. Using antibiotics indiscriminately can be likened to using powerful ammunition to kill a mouse, leaving one with no defense when a tiger threatens one's life.

Another example of public-scientist confrontation on the basis of knowledge is the controversy over laetrile. Although almost without exception the medical community rejects laetrile, putting it in the category of a "quack medicine" which may endanger the lives of those who use it in cancer therapy, public demand has resulted in specific legislation to legalize its use. This process is contrary to the regulatory powers of the Food and Drug Administration, which requires that a new drug be proven effective without serious side effects before it can be marketed for general use.

Value Systems

There is no aspect of life in which the value systems of the individual and society do not have profound, though at times subtle, effect. The smoker continues to smoke largely because, perhaps unconsciously, he or she has made a decision about the risks in terms of personal values; a higher value is placed on the immediate satisfactions of smoking than on the long-term preservation of health. Or such a person may reason that many daily activities, such as crossing the street, involve risks to one's well-being, and force a choice of relative risks, assigning an order value to them in terms of probability.

American society, with its current affluence and levels of achievement, values health as a right, not a luxury. This is reflected in the political arena, and in the increasing legislation ranging from Medicare to programs aimed at providing the means to achieve a high level of health and well-being. In addition, vast sums of money are being spent in the pursuit of better health. Factors influencing increased spending on health services include a public educated to be health service consumers and their willingness to spend, the increasing numbers of health service personnel, and the development of a wide variety of complex instruments that facilitate health care.

Attitudes toward the use of health care by the disadvantaged and poor are gradually changing, due in part to efforts to increase access to medical services. However, discrepancies remain. Too often, people living in ghetto areas have encountered cynicism, carelessness, rebuff, and assembly-line care from health services personnel. Figures 1-1, 1-2, and 1-3 illustrate these points. Figure 1-1 shows that the lowest income families were five times more likely than the highest income families to judge their health as only fair or poor. Even within the same income categories, racial minorities

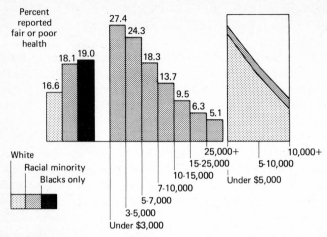

Figure 1-1 Assessment of health status. *(Source: USPHS National Center for Health Statistics, unpublished data. Health Interview Survey. Published in* Health of the Disadvantaged: Chart Book, *Department of Health Education and Welfare, Public Health Service, Health Resources Administration, Office of Health Resources Opportunity. DHEW publication No. (HRA) 77-628. September 1977, p. 18.)*

were still more likely than whites to judge their health as only fair or poor. With the introduction of Medicaid and Medicare, increased access to medical services has been helpful, as shown in Figure 1-2. Figure 1-3 shows that racial minorities and those below the near poverty level had significantly more waiting time at their regular source of care.

Table 1-1 illustrates the differences in expenditures for all personal health services by selected characteristics and source of payment, which reflect the impact of financial aspects on the use of health care services.

Changing Character of the Population

Simmons[15] has cited two characteristics of modern society which affect health care expectations and accomplishments: mobility (both lateral and vertical) and widespread understanding of its purposes, processes, and personnel. The mobility of which Simmons speaks is both literal, in the sense of moving from one location to another and figurative, in the movement from one social stratum to another. The latter movement may be up or down, with consequences directly proportional to the direction, i.e., the higher the social stratum, the greater the use of and expectations from health services. Implicit in the freedom of people to move—sometimes great distances between the states—is the continuing expectation that what they have become accustomed to in their original locations, they will find in the new. With the large number of families changing residence, similar standards of practice are developing in response to the expectations and demands of the people. More uniformity may be anticipated as fuller use of medical communications, information storage, and retrieval systems is made with the help of computers.

Related to population changes is the distribution of disease

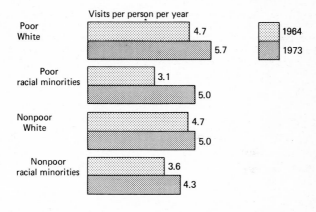

Note: The definition of poor and nonpoor is based on family income:

	Poor	Nonpoor
1964	under $3000	$3000 or over
1973	under $6000	$6000 or over

Figure 1-2 Doctor visits per person, 1964–1973. *(Source: Ronald W. Wilson and E. L. White: "Changes in Morbidity, Disability and Utilization Differentials between the Poor and Nonpoor: Data from the Health Interview Survey, 1964 and 1973." Paper given at the annual American Public Health Association meeting, 1974. Reprinted in* Health of the Disadvantaged: Chart Book, DHEW, PHS, Health Resources Administration, Office of Health Resources Opportunity. DHEW publication No. (HRA) 77-628. September 1977, p. 37.)

Office waiting time at regular source of care
by family income and by race: U. S. 1970

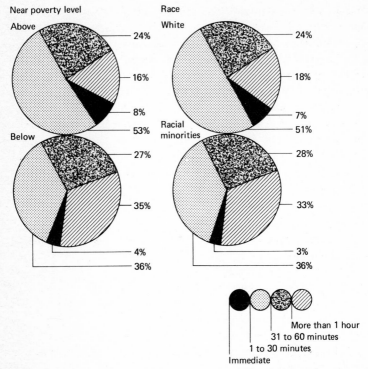

Figure 1-3 Office waiting time. *(Source: Lu Ann Aday and Ronald Anderson: "Development of Indices of Access to Medical Care," Health Administration Press, University of Michigan, 1974. Reprinted in* Health of the Disadvantaged: Chart Book, *DHEW, PHS, Health Resources Administration, Office of Health Resources Opportunity. DHEW publication No. (HRA) 77-628. September 1977, p. 37.)*

types and incidence. With more persons in the sixty-five-or-older bracket, more of the chronic, degenerative types of disease become prevalent. In contrast, the younger population is more vulnerable to acute infectious disease.

The stratification of the general populace into groups having social, economic, or political characteristics and goals has created various pressures on and for medical care. These pressure groups include, for example, professionals in health care organizations, labor unions, and government bureaucracies, each with its own concept of the quality, kind, and quantity of health care to be delivered.

The increase of "third party" agents involved in health insurance has made them effective in determining the quality of the services offered and the level of health benefits derived, since they are keenly interested in spending the money well.

Significant influences on health services are to be seen in federal programs, such as Medicare; professional education programs; licensure; consumer education; and the group efforts of the programs of voluntary health organizations and health agencies.

Research and Growing Knowledge

The expression "knowledge explosion" has become a cliché, yet there seems no other way to express the impact of scientific investigation on today's health care. This process is aided, and supports the implementation of its gains, by greater precision and sensitivity of the instruments used in research and practice.

The most formidable effect of the knowledge explosion is the rapid obsolescence not only of equipment but also of practitioners. Almost as formidable is the fragmentation of practice into specialties.

Specialization continues to stimulate the development of new, allied health professions as well as encouraging the growth of those already established. The complexity of health care demands the collaboration of specialized groups if it is to have quality and, remain individual and comprehensive. Progress toward "the greater medical profession" that Fox[3] proposes in the merger of physicians with other health professionals is not proceeding as rapidly as had been hoped, but is certainly a trend that is to be encouraged. The push toward comprehensive health care can be an important influence on collaboration, as is recognized by Wolf and Darley[17] in their definition of comprehensive care as "a system of person- and family-centered service, rendered by a well-balanced well-organized core of professional, technical, and vocational personnel who, by using facilities and equipment that are physically and

Table 1-1 Expenditures for Personal Health Services

Characteristic	Medicaid, welfare, free institution	Other free care	Source of payment Medicare	Voluntary insurance	Out-of-pocket	Other nonfree care	Total mean expenditures per person
Sex							
Male	$ 36	$ 14	$ 19	$ 66	$ 98	$1	$ 234
Female	26	2	22	85	119	4	258
Age							
0–5	12	a	—	69	54	1	135
6–17	14	2	—	31	63	1	110
18–34	74	10	—	88	117	8	296
35–54	20	13	—	82	121	a	236
55–64	23	10	a	211	197	4	445
65 and over	26	13	204	32	153	a	428
Poverty level							
Above near poverty	23	8	14	88	120	3	256
Below near poverty	57	8	42	34	70	2	213
Family income							
Under $2,000	88	9	83	23	98	1	302
$2,000–3,499	63	13	63	28	90	2	259
3,500–4,999	32	9	29	73	111	1	256
5,000–7,499	23	12	30	83	105	2	255
7,500–9,999	10	8	5	74	89	2	186
10,000–14,999	50	7	11	75	104	5	252
15,000 and over	5	4	6	103	140	2	260

Race							
White	29	8	21	81	116	3	258
Racial minority	45	8	15	40	53	2	162
Education of head							
8 years or less	32	11	42	52	96	1	234
9–11 years	22	4	20	55	89	2	193
12 years	56	5	14	75	98	2	249
13 years or more	9	11	9	116	146	5	295

Best estimate expenditures by selected characteristics and source of payment: 1970.

a = less than 50¢.

Source: Reprinted with permission from "Two Decades of Health Services," Ronald Andersen, Odin Anderson, and Joanna Lion, Ballinger Publishing Co., 1976, pp. 248–49, reprinted in *Health of the Disadvantaged: Chart Book*, DHEW, PHS, Health Resources Administration, Office of Health Resource Opportunity, DHEW publication no. (HRA) 77–628, September 1977, p. 97.

Table 1-2 Age of Population, Percent Distribution, and Rate of Change

Age	Population (in thousands)			Percent distribution				Change, 1970-75	
	1960	1970	1975	1960	1970	1975		Number	Percent
All Ages	180,671	204,335	213,631	100%	100%	100%		+9,297	+ 4.5%
Under 5 yrs.	20,341	17,163	15,896	11.3	8.4	7.4		-1,267	- 7.4
5 to 13 yrs.	32,965	36,675	44,456	18.2	17.9	15.7		-3,218	- 8.8
14 to 17 yrs.	11,219	15,854	16,943	6.2	7.8	7.9		+1,089	+ 6.9
18 to 24 yrs.	16,128	24,455	27,623	8.9	12.0	12.9		+3,168	+13.0
25 to 34 yrs.	22,919	25,146	30,936	12.7	12.3	14.5		+5,790	+23.0
35 to 44 yrs.	24,221	23,214	22,825	13.4	11.4	10.7		- 389	- 1.7
45 to 54 yrs.	20,578	23,254	23,772	11.4	11.4	11.1		+ 518	+ 2.2
55 to 64 yrs.	15,625	18,603	19,780	8.6	9.1	9.3		+1,177	+ 6.3
65 yrs. and over	16,675	19,972	22,400	9.2	9.8	10.5		+2,428	+12.2

Sources: Estimates of the Population of the United States, by Age, Sex, and Race: April 1, 1960 to July 1, 1974, *Current Population Reports* Series, no. 529, p. 25, September 1974:1; Estimates of the Population of the United States, by Age, Sex, and Race: 1970 to 1975, *Current Population Reports* Series no. 614, p. 25, December 1975:2.

functionally related, can deliver effective service at a cost that is economically compatible with individual, family, community, and national resources."

This definition also provides a statement of goals to be reached. Progress toward these goals is agonizingly slow because of the interaction of a variety of forces. For example, sheer size of the system, attitudes, the focus of education of health care personnel, and the necessity to set priorities that engage a wide spectrum of resources and energies are critical in order to move toward these goals, step by step.

PREVENTIVE HEALTH CARE

Attitudes of both the public and health care personnel are fundamental to the realization of the preventive maintenance aspects of health care. As Pelligrino points out, the public's order of concerns is with the availability of care for emergencies, acute illness, and easing of chronic illness. The types of care required to prevent illness and injury do not hold sufficiently high priority to influence practices to a very significant degree.

For the public, this apparent lack of concern may be due to the difficulty of dealing with a matter that involves benefits that are realized in the long term. Whether actually considered or not, the question seems to be "why bother with preventive care now, when there is no immediate benefit?" This leads to taking risks, and implies an assumption that curative health care will solve any problems that might arise years later.

Education of most health care personnel focuses on the diagnostic and curative aspects of health care. Preventive health maintenance aspects are, more than one wants to admit, almost incidental. In practice, the obvious needs of patients and clients for care of emergencies and acute illness naturally direct attention and efforts away from preventive care. This same focus of attention to curative medicine is also seen when there are little or no prospects for the patient's recovery. When faced with this situation, many physicians are at a loss because success is closely associated with *doing something* that results in recovery, yet the patient's need is for support. This is summarized in the statement "don't just do something;

stand there." Until the rewards and satisfactions of preventive maintenance are as highly valued as acute care, there is unlikely to be a shift in attitudes or education.

Pellegrino[11] defines health maintenance as sustaining, preserving, and supporting the individual's position in the health continuum, and involves both preventive and curative aspects. The objective of curative medicine is to bring the person back to the previous position on the continuum, with the possibility of improving that position. The objectives of preventive medicine are to avoid incidence of illness, and to interrupt progression of existing illness through intervention before the fact. Pellegrino's definition is elaborated further by the identification of three components: containment and easing existing chronic disease, detection of unsuspected disease that can be treated effectively at an early stage, and primary prevention. From the personnel standpoint, modifications in education and utilization of health care manpower within the framework of these three components appear to hold the best promise of success in reaching the goals of comprehensive care as a practice.

PERSONAL AND SOCIETAL ROLES IN HEALTH

The ultimate responsibility for health is an individual matter, yet is subject to the impacts of a wide range of influences. The issues are summarized with a high sense of urgency by Dr. John Knowles. Under the title of "Responsibility for Health," he writes:

> Most individuals do not worry about their health until they lose it. Uncertain attempts at healthy living may be thwarted by the temptations of a culture whose economy depends on high production and high consumption. Asceticism is reserved for hairshirted clerics and constipated cranks, and every time one of them dies at the age of 50, the hedonist smiles, inhales deeply, and takes another drink.
>
> Prevention of disease means forsaking the bad habits which many people enjoy—overeating, too much drinking, taking pills, staying up at night, engaging in promiscuous sex, driving too fast, and smoking cigarettes—or, put another way, it means doing things which require special effort—exercising regularly, improving nutrition, going to the dentist, practicing contraception, ensuring harmonious family life, submitting to screening examinations. The idea of individ-

ual responsibility flies in the face of American history, which has seen a people steadfastly sanctifying individual freedom while progressively narrowing it through the development of the beneficent state. On the one hand, social Darwinism maintains its hold on the American mind despite the best intentions of the neoliberals. Those who are not supine before the federal Leviathan proclaim the survival of the fittest. On the other, the idea of individual responsibility has given way to that of individual rights—or demands, to be guaranteed by government and delivered by public and private institutions. The cost of private excess is now a national, not an individual, responsibility. This is justified as individual freedom—but one man's freedom in health is another man's shackle in taxes and insurance premiums. I believe the idea of a "right" to health should be replaced by that of a moral obligation to preserve one's own health. The individual then has the "right" to expect help with information, accessible services of good quality, and minimal financial barriers. Meanwhile, the people have been led to believe that national health insurance, more doctors, and greater use of high-cost, hospital-based technologies will improve health. Unfortunately, none of them will.

The barriers to the assumption of responsibility for one's own health are lack of knowledge (implicating the inadequacies of formal education, the too-powerful force of advertising, and the informal systems of continuing education), lack of sufficient interest in and knowledge about what is preventable and the cost/benefit ratios of nationwide health programs (implicating the powerful interests in the health establishment, which could not be less interested, and calling for a much larger investment in fundamental and applied research), and a culture which has progressively eroded the idea of individual responsibility while stressing individual rights, the responsibility of society at large, and the steady growth of production and consumption ("We have met the enemy and he is us!").

The individual must realize that perpetuating the present system of high-cost, after-the-fact medicine will only result in higher costs and greater frustration. The next major advances in the health of the American people will be determined by what the individual is willing to do for himself and for society at large. If he is willing to follow reasonable rules for healthy living, he can extend his life and enhance his own and the nation's productivity. If he is willing to reassert his authority with his children, he can provide for their optimal mental and physical development. If he participates fully in private and public efforts to reduce the hazards of the environment, he can reduce the causes of premature death and disability. If he is unwilling to do these things, he should stop complaining about the rising costs of medical care and the disproportionate share of the gross national product that is consumed by health care. He can either remain the problem or become the solution to it; beneficent government cannot.*

REFERENCES

1 "The American Health Empire: Power, Profits, and Politics," A report from the Health Policy Advisory Center, Vintage Books, New York, 1971.

2 Claiborne, Robert, The great health care rip-off, *Saturday Review,* 7 Jan. '78, pp. 10–16, 50.

3 Fox, T. F., The Greater Medical Profession, *Lancet,* 271:779, 1956.

4 Guyton, A. C., "Functions of the Human Body," 2d ed., W. B. Saunders Company, Philadelphia, 1964, p. 4.

5 Illich, I., "Medical Nemesis: the Expropriation of Health," Calder and Boyars, London, 1975.

6 Kennedy, Edward M., "In Critical Condtion: The Crisis in America's Health Care," Simon & Schuster Inc., New York, 1972.

7 Kunnes, Richard, "Your Money or Your Life," Dodd, Mead & Company, Inc. New York, 1971.

8 Lenihan, J., and W. W. Fletcher (eds.), "Health and the Environment," Blackie & Son, Ltd., Glasgow, 1976.

9 McKeown, A., "The Role of Medicine: Dream, Mirage, or Nemesis?" Nuffield Provincial Hospitals Trust, London, 1976.

10 Merton, Robert, Issues in Growth of a Profession, in *Proceedings of the 41st Annual Convention of the American Nursing Association,* Atlantic City, N.J., June 10, 1958, p. 302.

11 Pellegrino, Edmund, Preventive Care and the Allied Health Professions, in "Review of Allied Health Education, 1," Joseph Hamburg (ed.), University Press of Kentucky, Lexington, 1974, pp. 1–18.

12 Pyle, Howard, The Secret Reasons People Won't Buy Seat Belts, *Home and Highway,* **13**:17–19, Autumn 1964, Publication of Allstate Insurance Co., Skokie, Ill.

---

*John Knowles, President, Rockefeller Foundation. Editorial in *Science,* 198: 1106, Dec. 16, 1977. Adapted from his article in *Daedalus,* 106:57; reprinted in *Doing Better and Feeling Worse: Health in the United States.* Norton, New York, 1977, p. 57. Copyright 1977 by the American Association for the Advancement of Science.

13 Schopenhauer, A., "Studies in Pessimism: Further Psychological Observations," Modern Library, Inc., New York, p. 77.

14 Selye, Hans, "The Stress of Life," McGraw-Hill Book Company, New York, 1966.

15 Simmons, Leo W., Change in the Social Order as It Affects Health Service, *Hosp. Progr.* **45:**81–86, June 1964.

16 Sinacore, J. S., "Health: A Quality of Life," The Macmillan Company, New York, 1974.

17 Wolf, S. G. Jr., and W. Darley, Medical Education and Practice: Relationships and Responsibilities in a Changing Society, *J. Med. Educ.* **40:**387–389, part 2, 1965.

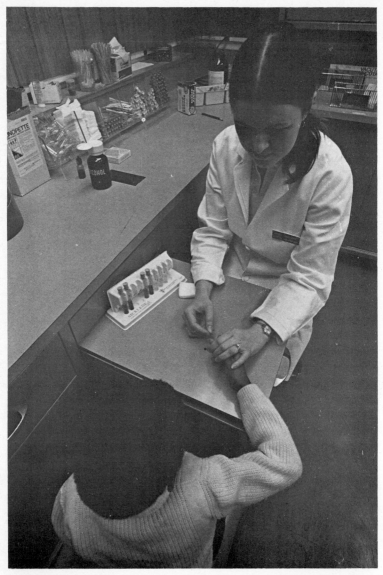

Compassion and cooperation combine for the patient's benefit. *(Courtesy of Bill Rogers.)*

2
THE PATIENT

Language reflects many of our perceptions of our world. For example, our word for the person who is ill, patient, stems from the Latin *pati,* meaning to suffer, and our word for the person who is in need is client, derived from the Latin *clinare,* to lean. In each instance, it is easy to trace how these words developed their modern meanings, for indeed illness does frequently involve suffering, and need stemming from some kind of loss does necessitate the support of another person. Both terms are common in health care.

HISTORICAL PERSPECTIVE

We have come to expect certain behavior of the patient and the client. These expectations have slowly emerged from the sociological and religious aspects of our culture, independent of a strictly medical view.

At the most primitive cultural level, the sick person was left to fend for himself or die; the well had no obligation to assist him.

The objective was to rid the group of a detrimental, hindering element. Complete isolation from society was the lot of one who fell ill; there was no attempt to ascertain causes and cures of illness.

Still at the primitive level, but somewhat more advanced, was (and is yet) the concept of illness being caused by an evil spirit or the curse of a malignant person. In either case, the tribe then felt a responsibility to the sick person, who was considered a victim, in need of incantations to appease the evil spirits or of a countercurse to negate the power of the person inflicting the disease.

The Old Testament is studded with references to illness as punishment for sin—the patient's own sin, or the sins of his family. This is a reflection of the characterization of a vengeful, harsh God whose justice demanded "an eye for an eye and a tooth for a tooth" kind of retribution for breaking His laws. Illness and suffering were also considered, much in the same light, as expiation for sin.

A sharp contrast appears in the New Testament references to illness. The Christian ethos made possible a positive approach to suffering, viewing it as a means of grace that freed a person from the stigma of sin. In fact, disease came to be seen as grace, and the healthy could participate in such grace by associating with the sick. Caring for the sick became an obligation for the Christian. And in the East, Buddhism was also teaching compassion for the ill. The patient was no longer an outcast.

In ancient Greece, health was regarded as one of the highest values. Conversely, disease was an evil in that it rendered a person unworthy. The stigma of unworthiness was to be avoided, as any degrading condition would be. The sense of unworthiness associated with disease made a deep impression in its time, and has ever since.

Modern Developments

Secular authority became influential in health care during the eighteenth and nineteenth centuries, and, as it formed the ideals of the common good of the whole people, "contributions to the care of the sick grew richer and larger, finding in the course of time, social security as its most striking expression."[19]

Today, despite the general wish to help the patient, some remnants of the old concepts—primitive, Old Testament, and ancient

Greek—are still with us, submerged in the subconscious desire to get away from sickness and disease. Illness as punishment for sin is an idea still current in some modern cultures. The same idea is exemplified as well in the self-punishment that is sometimes manifested in mental illness. The ancients judged the sick as lesser people; that judgment, again usually a subconscious one, is often applied to crippled persons, and calls for conscious effort to resist impulsive actions that might easily hurt them psychologically.

As Sigerist[19] points out, the fact of illness, no matter to what degree, interrupts the rhythm of life, isolates the sick person from others, calls for passivity (another definition of "patient"), and may bring discomfort and pain, the pain inducing fear.

THE SICK ROLE

Parsons[17] has characterized the sick role as having two rights and two duties. The rights are freedom from blame and exemption from normal roles and task obligations. These rights are, however, socially legitimate only partially and conditionally. Their limits are defined in the duties: to do everything possible to recover and, in so doing, to seek technically competent help.

Abuse of the rights and negligence of the duties are sometimes seen. For example, the patient may unconsciously seek release from responsibility by hypochondriasis or by frankly feigning illness. Refusal to seek competent technical aid or to follow recommendations for treatment may be due to deep-seated fear or contempt. Whatever the reasons for such deviant behavior, patients should be helped to view their behavior realistically.

A delicate balance of roles must be maintained in the world of those institutions offering care for the sick—the patient vis-à-vis those who care for the patient. Main[16] has pointed this up very well:

> The concept of a hospital as a refuge too often means that patients are robbed of their status as human beings. Too often they are called "good" or "bad" only according to the degree of their passivity in the face of the hospital demand for their obedience, dependence, and gratitude. The fine traditional mixture of charity and discipline they receive is a practiced technique for removing their initiative as adult

beings and making them "patients." They are then less trouble for the staff.

PSYCHOLOGIC ASPECTS OF ILLNESS

Self-Concept

The patient's self-concept, particularly in relation to serious illness, is an important determinant of responses to such a crisis. Because each person is a complex of elements long in the making—some culturally imbued, others the product of experience and personality—reactions cannot be predicted. One person may respond to illness as a form of martyrdom and see himself as suffering for others. Another may see herself as having privileged status and act this out in demanding behavior.

Self-concept also influences the patient's response to a treatment regimen. For example, a husky, vigorous man, an "outdoors type," may see himself as too strong to be ill, too masculine to depend on others to take care of his daily needs. Consider the affront to his concept of basic autonomy if his illness is such that he cannot feed himself. Accustomed to physical activity, he finds it extremely difficult to channel his activity-oriented energies to quieter levels, yet he must. Perhaps his latent evaluation of illness is that it makes him unworthy, and if so, he may at first demonstrate a will to deny it, and then to expend effort to recover. Being aware of how patients see themselves is of great importance in planning their care, making it possible to take advantage of the positive aspects and, at the same time, reducing the stress of the negative aspects. The health professional and the patient can then work together for the patient's benefit.

Stages of Reaction to Illness

Usually the first reaction to illness is to deny its presence, or to explain it away in terms of the known, the trivial, or the familiar. The pain radiating to the arm in myocardial infarct may be "explained" as arthritis and treated as such. Epigastric distress may be attributed to injudicious eating and treated with an antacid. When it finally becomes too obvious to deny and is resistant to ordinary remedies, the patient sees illness as a reality, and, depending on its severity, there is a sense of loss and a threat because of reduced functional ability.

Dependency is the hallmark of the acute stage of illness—imposed by the patient's incapacity and by the very real demands of those who provide the care. Some patients may have a psychological need for succor which may prove an obstacle to recovery. Dependency is a form of regression to childhood and may be manifested in several ways. Egocentricity—witness the dominating, intolerant, demanding sickroom despot—is a familiar pattern. Regression may also cause a lowering of emotional control so that there are exaggerated reactions to ordinary stimuli, accompanied by a need for help, attention, and affection. With this type of reaction, the patient may shift roles from adult to child. The physician's role then becomes that of surrogate father, the nurse's that of surrogate mother.

When patients begin to convalesce, the shift back to adult responsibility and autonomy occurs, preparing them for a return to the normal routines of life when they are well.

This simplified tracing of the stages of illness is subject to the pitfalls of any generalization. However, it is a fact that reactions to illness are based on complex mechanisms which affect the patient's way of coping with fear, anxieties about possible mutilation, and reduced ability to function.

The fact of being ill interposes complications which must be dealt with just as carefully as those that precipitate and cause the illness; otherwise, medical services may not be successful in returning the patient to productive life. Illness may provide the patient an opportunity to gratify an aggressive need to control others, and thus might negate many of the attempts to serve medical needs. The patient's need for independence and autonomy may be revealed by a generally disagreeable disposition, a disregard for medical advice and control. These manifestations are of great importance to those who work with the patient on a one-to-one basis, and must be considered in planning and carrying out a therapeutic program.

The Family's Response to Illness

One difficulty for the family caring for one of its members is balancing the support and the discipline required in any regimen of treatment. An example of the interaction between a young husband and wife may make this point clear. The wife, a victim of multiple sclerosis, was angry and resentful because her husband would not acquiesce to her every wish nor anticipate all her needs for assistance. When she expressed her feelings, her husband's response was that he did not do all she wanted him to do because that would have reduced her capacity for self-help even more. Happily, the wife saw the wisdom of his so-called neglect, and grew better able to do for herself than she had thought possible.

The whole family may be affected by one member's illness if that illness deprives the patient of the usual roles. If the father is the focus of all work responsibility, authority, and decision-making, any event that curtails his function in these roles can result in problems. Traditionally considered "the heart of home," the mother's absence or incapacity may bankrupt family resources for its usual emotional support and affection. Shared emotional support and affection among members of the family create a better situation in any case.

In the presence of chronic illness or one, like cancer, in which the outcome is predictable but may extend over a relatively long period of time, the family of the patient may also become drained emotionally and physically. Fatigue may lead to withdrawal of support at most, or episodes of impatience at the least. When this occurs, the patient may believe that he is a nuisance. Dorroh[7] quotes a patient's description of this situation for one who had cancer: "At first my family and my friends crowded around and tried to do everything they could, but after a while, my friends began to come around less often and my family seemed bored. I don't think my family ever wished me dead, but they acted as if my illness were a nuisance. I felt the same way about myself." Patience and attention to even the smallest manifestation of love and caring for the individual assume great importance, and cannot be taken for granted.

Response of Health Care Personnel to Illness
Persons who choose to serve the needs of the ill must recognize at the outset that they will be an integral part of the reactions that occur, and must be prepared to deal not only with the responses of

others, but with their own feelings as well. We may be very well prepared to deal with these matters on a detached, "intellectual" level, but find our feelings get in the way. Generous measures of understanding and self-discipline are necessary for anyone who serves the needs of those who are ill. One must understand oneself, why certain things and people evoke certain types of reactions, and discipline oneself to focus on what needs to be done to offer the best help to patients. The extremes of too much or too little sympathy are common problems. There may also be occasions when anger is roused, or persons or certain types of illnesses provoke dislike. Particular sensitivity is required to avoid falling into the trap of superiority or power, for those who care for the sick are frequently decision makers who "control" the patient.

SOCIOLOGIC ASPECTS OF ILLNESS

Individual and social reactions to illness do not exist apart from each other. As medical science developed more skill and knowledge in diagnosing and treating disease, as well as in preventing it, some of the purely medical pressures have been relieved. As a consequence, there has been a great deal more research applied to medical sociology, giving us better insight into some of the vexing problems involved in illness. By their very nature, imbedded as they are in the fabric of culture, the elements of these problems are not easily teased out for inspection. However, some general guidelines are clear, and must be used if long-term preventive measures are to be successful. One of the best discussions of this entire subject is that of Esther Lucile Brown.[4]

Each individual is a part of a culture which includes customs, traditions, values, patterns of interaction, methods of economic support, and techniques for both positive and negative controls on the members of the culture. In an example cited by Brown, the cultural influence on a patient's expectations is clear.

A Polish-American patient, who was suffering from intractable pain, had taken it for granted that if he were very sick he would be given massive doses of individualized attention, including a nurse's hand on his forehead or an arm around his shoulder. (Although he was born in the United States, this expectation was apparently in accord with practices in the part of the country from which his parents had come.) When he received no such attention in the particular hospital, he concluded that all the staff disliked him. As a result, said he to the social scientist interviewing him, he knew his discomfort was much worse than it would have been otherwise. When the interviewer reported what he had learned, the doctors and nurses were amazed and distressed. They decided they did not know how to give the kind of care the patient wanted and hence had him transferred to the psychiatric service in the hope that the staff there would be able to do better. For this patient, who already felt rejected, the transferral must have seemed like the final act of rejection!

Culture influences the types and incidence of diseases, as well as the reactions of the sick individual. The relationship between culture and disease is sometimes obvious, as in diseases triggered by a lack of essential foods—such as proteins—or an excess of certain kinds of foods. These nutritional factors result in making the members of the given culture vulnerable to diseases having their roots in dietary habits. However, cultural taboos are generally indirect in their relationship to disease. For example, venereal diseases can be controlled only if the public is fully informed about the transmission of these diseases, their symptomatology, and the availability of treatment. The Victorian suppression of sex information long impeded efforts to control venereal disease; but attitudes about sex have been changing. Now that the cultural taboo has been breached, public health authorities have been able to conduct public information campaigns as part of their attack on venereal diseases.

A telling example of the shift in attitudes and acceptability of discussion of venereal disease as a public health problem is the public television documentary on the subject, for which Dick Cavett was the host-narrator.

SOCIOECONOMIC FACTORS OF ILLNESS

Sometimes a duodenal ulcer is jokingly called a status symbol—a fairly accurate indication of the sufferer's place on the socioeconomic ladder, and the status-seeker's reward for his intensive drive to succeed in climbing higher. As with many jokes, there is an element of tragic truth in this one. In different strata of society certain diseases have a higher incidence. In part, this reflects the cultural expectations of members of each stratum; it also reflects the group's value attitudes toward seeking medical attention, and, in some instances, deprivation.

Tables 2-1 and 2-2, and Figure 2-1 reflect the shifts that have occurred in recent years in terms of utilization of health care services. These shifts probably represent increased accessibility because of the Medicare and Medicaid programs, for example. A

Table 2-1 Regular Source of Medical Care: 1963 and 1970

| | Source of regular care | | | | | | | |
| | Percent M.D. | | Percent clinic | | Percent osteopath, other | | Percent no regular care | |
Characteristic	1963	1970	1963	1970	1963	1970	1963	1970
Sex								
Male	71	65	11	18	5	4	14	13
Female	74	69	11	17	4	5	11	9
Age								
1–5	78	69	11	21	3	4	8	6
6–17	72	67	13	20	5	5	10	8
18–34	69	65	10	18	4	4	17	13
35–54	72	69	9	14	5	4	14	13
55–64	75	67	9	16	4	5	12	12
65 and over	75	69	9	16	3	4	13	11
Family income								
Low	63	56	17	24	4	4	16	16
Middle	75	68	10	17	4	5	11	10
High	75	74	7	14	6	4	12	8
Race								
White	74	69	9	16	5	5	12	10
Racial minority	62	51	20	30	3	3	15	16
Education of head								
Less than 9 yrs.	69	64	13	19	4	4	14	13
9–11 years	72	60	11	23	4	5	13	12
12 years	76	72	9	14	4	6	11	8
13 years or more	77	72	8	16	3	2	12	10

Source: R. Andersen, O. Anderson, and J. Lion, "Two Decades of Health Services," Ballinger Publishing Company, Cambridge, Mass., 1976, p. 17. Reprinted in *Health of the Disadvantaged: Chart Book,* DHEW PHS Health Resources Administration, Office of Health Resources Opportunity, DHEW publication no. (HRA) 77-628, September 1977.

Table 2-2   Number of Dental Visits per Year: 1975

Characteristic	All ages	Under 15 yrs.	15–44 yrs.	45–64 yrs.	65+ yrs.
Total	1.6	1.5	1.8	1.8	1.2
Male	1.5	1.4	1.6	1.6	1.4
Female	1.7	1.5	2.0	1.9	1.0
Race					
White	1.7	1.6	1.9	1.8	1.2
Racial minority	1.0	0.6	1.2	1.3	0.6
Black only	1.0	0.6	1.2	1.4	0.6
Income					
Under $3,000	1.1	0.8	1.4	1.2	0.6
$3,000–4,999	1.1	0.8	1.4	1.4	0.8
5,000–6,999	1.1	0.9	1.2	1.2	1.2
7,000–9,999	1.5	1.0	1.7	1.6	1.6
10,000–14,999	1.6	1.4	1.7	1.6	1.5
15,000–24,999	2.0	1.8	2.0	2.1	1.8
25,000+	2.6	2.6	2.6	2.5	2.4
Race and income					
White					
Under $5,000	1.2	1.1	1.6	1.3	1.2
$5,000–9,999	1.4	1.0	1.5	1.5	1.4
10,000+	2.0	1.9	2.0	2.1	1.8
Racial minority					
Under $5,000	0.8	0.4	0.9	1.4	*
$5,000–9,999	1.1	0.8	1.3	1.3	*
10,000+	1.2	0.8	1.4	1.3	*

Source: *Health of the Disadvantaged: Chart Book*, DHEW, PHS, Health Resources Administration, Office of Health Resources Opportunity, DHEW Publication no. (HRA) 77-628, September 1977.

comparison of the number of visits per year by minorities indicates that there was a slightly higher average for them, which suggests that they delay seeing a physician until the problem becomes more serious. A trend of interest in Table 2-1 is the increased use of clinics, which reflects their growth and accessibility.

Kandle[12] notes that the attention to chronic illness and its relationship to the physical and social environment is a good example of changing public health practice. He cites a special project carried out by St. Peter's Hospital, New Brunswick, N.J., and the state

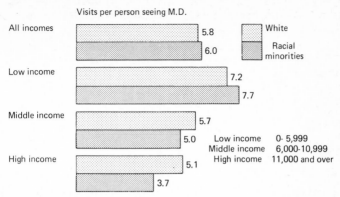

Figure 2-1 Doctor visits per patient. *(Source: R. Anderson, J. Lion, and O. Anderson, "Two Decades of Health Services," Ballinger Publishing Co., 1976. Reprinted in* Health of the Disadvantaged: Chart Book, *DHEW, PHS, Health Resources Administration, Office of Health Resources Opportunity. DHEW publication No. (HRA) 77-628. September 1977.)*

health department, which dealt primarily with congestive heart failure. The purpose of the project was "to mobilize community resources to keep these patients at home, to keep them functionally as well as possible, and to prevent previous need for rehospitalization and recurrence of congestive heart failure episodes." The study team found that half of the forty-six patients participating in the project had no family; only one person had an annual income of $4,000 and eight patients had less than half this amount. Their living quarters were below standard in many respects (for example, water being available only from a pump or tap in the yard).

Low income and poor housing go together. To the patient with congestive heart failure, they create special stresses. When the monthly income for food, rent, and clothing is $95, an expenditure of $20 for prescriptions can be catastrophic. As Kandle points out, "The stark reality of these facts are grim reminders that the social ills of these patients are as severe as the damage to their hearts. To treat their bodies only is clearly irresponsible."

MORTALITY

In all of our discussions up to this point, the assumption has been that the goal of medical service is to restore patients to at least their former level of health, or, if possible, to improve that level. It should not be the only assumption, however, for humankind is mortal, and it is just as important to consider what is involved when death is the outcome of an illness.

There are times when the fact of death's inevitability must be faced and decisions that may be excruciatingly difficult made. These are the times that call for all the mature inner resources of everyone concerned if the second goal of health care is to be accomplished: to provide, as nearly as possible, an environment for a dignified death, along with compassionate support to those who mourn that death.

The paradox involved in this aspect of medical service is a very real dilemma which may be expressed "I am bound, by my obligation to society, my profession, and humane instincts to assist in the preservation of life as far as possible. But the mere prolongation of this life by heroic measures is a prolongation of suffering." The critical point at issue comes with the recognition of the imminence of death. When death is imminent and inevitable, it is neither scientific nor humane to protract the life of the patient. Only when there is reasonable hope of sustaining life for more than a few days should every effort be made to delay death. Otherwise, life-preserving treatment ceases to be a gift and becomes a means of prolonging agony. The dignity of all persons and their right to live and die peacefully must be recognized.

Elisabeth Kübler-Ross was in the vanguard of those who have contributed first to sensitivity to problems of death and dying, then to supportive studies expanding on the subject, based on their own experience in treating patients. In her book *On Death and Dying*[15] she identifies five stages of reactions common to the process: denial, anger, bargaining, depression, and acceptance. These reactions are characterized by Dr. Kübler-Ross as "defense mechanisms in psychiatric terms, and coping mechanisms to deal with extremely difficult situations." She notes that their duration is variable, and sometimes concurrent, and that hope usually persists throughout all the stages.

Denial is the initial reaction typified by "no, not me; it can't be true." The denial associated with serious illness is, of course, more deeply felt than in other instances. *Anger* is not only difficult for the patient, but also for those in attendance, for "this anger is displaced in all directions and projected onto the environment at times almost at random." In effect, the patient is asking "why me?" *Bargaining* is a form of coping which involves postponement of the inevitable as a "prize" for doing what is expected—the childlike manner of being good. It also functions as a goal-directed form of coping, concentrating energy on what is perceived as an attainable objective, for example, the young wife who has been a significant contributor to her husband's work on his doctoral degree, and therefore "bargains" for time and the strength to attend the ceremony when he gets his degree. *Depression* comes with the realization of great losses, losses that come in a variety of forms. They may be, for example, physical when surgery is involved; financial, as is to be expected when treatment and hospitalization over long periods of time are required; or psychological, when there is diminished control. The depression of these cases falls within the category of "reactive depression," in contrast to "preparatory depression." The latter involves the depression associated with recognition of loss of loved objects. In working through this stage, the patient is preparing for the final stage—acceptance. *Acceptance* is not so much a matter of giving up as it is of acquiescence; it is being without fear and despair. The fear has been worked through in the first three stages; despair has been brought into balance by the mourning of "good grief" of the fourth stage. Acceptance is a time of relative peace and passivity, when support by gestures is more important than by words.

A PATIENT'S BILL OF RIGHTS

In December 1972, the American Hospital Association distributed a twelve-point statement "A Patient's Bill of Rights"* which was characterized in the cover letter to institutional members as "one of the most significant public documents ever developed by the American Hospital Association." This document was made public in January 1973. The rights enumerated seem so fundamental that it is not surprising that some responded with questions as to why it was necessary to promulgate them in this formal manner. One such

*See Appendix 1 for the full text.

response made in a national lay magazine editorial by Gaylin,[†] is critical of the fact that the Association addressed the problem from the patient's view, rather than cautioning hospitals about the violations of patients' rights ". . . some of which have the mandate of law, and warning them they must no longer presume on the innocence of their customers or the indifference of judicial authorities." Gaylin acknowledges this as a well-intentioned and ". . . a patently decent document . . .," but parries that with:

> In effect, all that the document does is return to the patient, with an air of largess, some of the rights hospitals have stolen from him. It is the thief lecturing his victim on self-protection—i.e., the hospital instructs the patient to make sure that the hospital treats him according to the rules of decency and law to which he is entitled.

The combination of the AHA document and Gaylin's critique has the potential for a salutary effect on health care personnel in hospitals, in the long run accomplishing the purposes of each, especially if brought to the attention of students preparing for careers serving patients. Certainly, the document provides a valuable summary of factors through which they can become acquainted with patients' rights and the corresponding responsibilities they must identify and assume as part of professional practice.

REFERENCES

1 Allport, Gordon, "The Nature of Prejudice," Doubleday & Company, Inc., Garden City, N.Y., 1958.

2 Areng, C. D., Sympathy and Empathy, *J.A.M.A.*, **167**:448–452, May 24, 1958.

3 Brim, O. G., H. E. Freeman, S. Levine, and N. A. Scotch (eds.), "The Dying Patient," Russell Sage Foundation, New York, 1964.

4 Brown, Esther Lucile, "Newer Dimensions of Patient Care: Patients as People," Russell Sage Foundation, New York, 1964.

5 Cobb, B., et al., Patient-responsible Delay of Treatment in Cancer: Social Psychological Study, *Cancer*, **7**:920–926, September 1954.

6 Connally, Grace, What Acceptance Means of Patients, *Am. J. Nurs.*, **60**:1754–1757, December 1960.

[†]Willard Gaylin, "The Patient's Bill of Rights," editorial in *Saturday Review,* Mar. 10, 1973, p. 22.

7   Dorroh, Thelma L., "Between Patient and Health Worker," McGraw-Hill Book Company, New York, 1974.

8   Duff, R. S., and A. B. Hollingshead, "Sickness and Society," Harper & Row, Publishers, Inc., New York, 1968.

9   Etzwiler, D. D., Why Not Put Your Patients under Contract, *Prism*, **2:**126–128, January 1974.

10 Glaser, B. G., and A. L. Strauss, "Time for Dying," Aldine Publishing Company, Chicago, 1968.

11 Highley, Betty, and Catherine Norris, When a Student Dislikes a Patient, *Am. J. Nurs.*, **57:**1163–1166, September 1957.

12 Kandle, R. P., Changing Times in Public Health, Paper read at a colloquium on Planning for Future Medical Care, Academy of Medicine, New Brunswick, N.J., Oct. 14, 1965.

13 King, Stanley H., Social Psychological Factors in Illness, in H. E. Freeman, Sol Levine, and L. G. Reeder (eds.), "Handbook of Medical Sociology," Prentice-Hall, Inc., Englewood Cliffs, N.J. 1963, pp. 99–121.

14 Knowles, John H., "Doing Better and Feeling Worse: Health in the United States," W.W. Norton & Company, Inc., New York, 1977.

15 Kübler-Ross, Elisabeth, "On Death and Dying," Macmillan Publishing Company, Inc., New York, 1973.

16 Main, T. F., The Hospital as a Therapeutic Institution, *Bull, Menninger Clinic,* **X:**66–70, 1946.

17 Parsons, Talcott, Definitions of Health and Illness in the Light of American Values and Social Structure, in E. G. Jaco (ed.), "Patients, Physicians and Illness," The Free Press of Glencoe, New York, 1959, pp. 165–187.

18 Ramsey, P., "The Patient as a Person," Yale University Press, New Haven, Conn., 1970.

19 Roemer, M. I. (ed.), "Henry E. Sigerist on the Sociology of Medicine," MD Publications, Inc., New York, 1960, pp. 9–22.

20 WHO, "Health Aspects of Human Rights," Geneva, 1976.

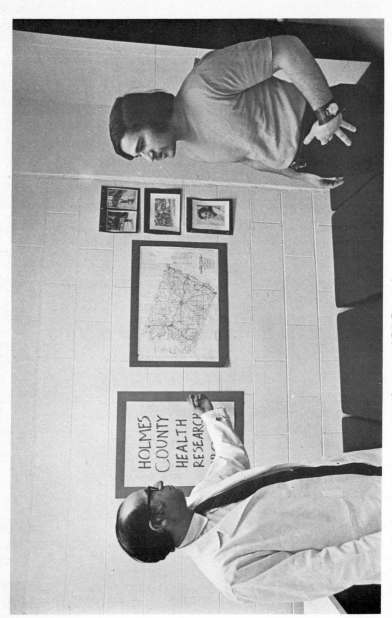

Health begins in plans for the community. *(Courtesy of Bill Rogers.)*

3

AGENCIES FOR HEALTH CARE

GENERAL CONSIDERATIONS

One of the hallmarks of American society is its organizations. These range from simple local club-type organizations to complex business organizations, the giants of industry. All are cooperative systems adaptive to social structures made up of interacting individuals, subgroups, and both formal and informal relationships. Cooperative systems or organizations depend on the balancing influence of both internal and external factors which act upon them—in reaching decisions, taking action, and making adjustments. These are the necessary functions of the organization if it is to achieve its stated goals, and they represent its conscious attempts to mobilize available resources for that achievement. Authority within the organization emphasizes factors of cohesion and persuasion to focus upon the accomplishments which the organization has chosen to make.

Health care in America is big business. As a business it is organized in a variety of ways, each pattern dictated by goals which serve some segment of the health field. The multiplicity of these health organizations, or agencies is a reflection of the complexity of the field. No one organization or agency is capable of dealing with all the elements of health care, nor should it be expected to. Thus multiplicity of agencies also demonstrates the tremendous growth of knowledge and the increasing sensitivity of society to the needs of its people. In turn, the people are being educated to recognize needs that may not be apparent to them but are nonetheless real.

Agencies for health care may be classified as government, voluntary, and institutional, but they are not limited in scope, for there are overlapping areas. For example, government agencies include regulatory bodies such as the Division of Biologics Standards and the Food and Drug Administration; and institutional agencies such as the Veterans Administration hospitals. A primary concern is that all of these agencies for health care cooperate and do their best to coordinate their efforts toward achieving specific goals. The dynamic character of interaction and mutual impact calls for these agencies to participate still more in coordinating efforts if health care is to improve to the extent hoped for at costs that are manageable. Unfortunately, the nature of organizations as social entities with their built-in proclivities for perpetuation and "empire building" and the sheer numbers of programs are the most potent forces countering cooperation and coordination.

WORLD HEALTH ORGANIZATION

While not strictly an agency of a government, for the United Nations is its parent, the World Health Organization (WHO) may be considered a government agency in that its programs are carried out through the cooperation of the governments of participating nations. Established in 1948, the World Health Organization is a specialized agency of the United Nations charged with furthering international cooperation for improvement of conditions of health throughout the world. Two other large-scale health organizations had been created, and abandoned, earlier in the century. The International Office of Public Health, with headquarters in Paris, was established in 1907. The League of Nations also had a division of health, which was established in 1923. From each of these organizations WHO inherited various programs related to epidemic control, quarantine, and measurement and standardization of drugs. But under its constitution, WHO was given a much broader mandate: to promote the attainment of the "highest possible level of health" by all peoples. In the constitution, health is defined positively as "a state of complete mental, physical, and social well-being and not merely the absence of disease or infirmity." It goes on to say that "good health is held to be fundamental to world peace and security."

The international headquarters of WHO is located in Geneva, Switzerland. The staff includes more than one thousand persons representing fifty nationalities. To accomplish its goals, three major functions have been identified: to be a central clearing house for information and research services; to establish measures for control of epidemic and endemic diseases; and to strengthen and expand the public health administrations of member nations. The third function listed is considered the most important task of WHO.

As a clearinghouse, there are a number of subsidiary functions related to information and research services. These include:

1 Publicizing international sanitary regulations
2 Dissemination of information about incidences of pestilential diseases
3 Publishing and distributing information to keep all national health administration up to date regarding new techniques and drugs

In its efforts to control epidemic and endemic diseases, WHO promotes mass campaigns involving:

1 Vaccination programs
2 Instruction in the use of antibiotics and insecticides
3 Establishment of local health centers
4 Aid in the development of national training institutes for health personnel
5 Teachers for short-course training experiments

6   Traveling fellowship awards to health administrators, nurses, and technologists

In a typical year, WHO is involved in 700 health projects distributed among more than a hundred countries and territories of the world.

FEDERAL AGENCIES

Congress

The story of federal agencies for health care begins with the Congress, which authorizes their establishment, often legislates particular programs and, of course, appropriates the funds to maintain them. Health-related concerns are the responsibility of three subcommittees of each of the houses of Congress, as shown in Table 3-1.

The legislative process involves a series of procedures before a bill becomes law. Under the supervision of the senator or representative, the bill is drafted by their respective staff members, often in collaboration between the senator and representative. The appropriate subcommittee conducts hearings and may modify the original draft of the bill. On approval by the subcommittee, the process of hearings and possible modifications is repeated by the full committee. On approval by the full committee, the bill begins its tortuous way through the parliamentary thickets of the Congress. Debate is conducted and frequently amendments are made. If the House and Senate bills emerge from this process with substantial differences, a House–Senate conference committee negotiates agreement, which is then voted on by the House and Senate. The bill then goes to the President, who may sign it into law, or veto it. If vetoed, a two-thirds majority of both houses of Congress is required for an override.

Cabinet Departments Concerned with Health Affairs

The Department of Health, Education and Welfare is, of course, the primary seat of federal activities in health affairs. However, as Table 3-2 shows, other departments and some independent agencies or entities are involved as well. Table 3-3 shows the Department of Health, Education and Welfare components in health affairs.

Table 3-1 Congressional Committees

	Committee	Subcommittee	Number of members, subcommittee*
Senate	Finance	Health	5 Democrats, 2 Republicans
	Human Resources	Health	8 Democrats, 3 Republicans
	Appropriations	HEW Appropriations	8 Democrats, 4 Republicans
House of Representatives	Ways and Means	Health	9 Democrats, 4 Republicans
	Interstate and Foreign Commerce	Health and Environment	10 Democrats, 4 Republicans
	Appropriations	HEW Appropriations	7 Democrats, 3 Republicans

*Note that since the Democrats control Congress, by virtue of being in the majority, they are also in the majority on committees and subcommittees, and hold the chairmanships.

Table 3-2   Federal Departments with Interests in Health Affairs

Department	Health-related component
Agriculture	Agriculture Research Service
	Food and Nutrition Service
Commerce	National Bureau of Standards
	Institute for Materials Research
	Bureau of the Census
	National Oceanic and Atmospheric Administration
Defense	University of Health Sciences
	Armed Forces Medical Units
Housing and Urban Development	Office of Environmental Quality
Justice	Drug Enforcement Administration
Labor	Occupational Safety and Health Administration
State	Office of Food for Peace
	Bureau for Population and Humanitarian Assistance
Energy	Division of Environment and Safety
	Biomedical and Environmental Research
	Operational Safety
	Reactor Safety
	Nuclear Regulations Commission
Independent Agencies and Entities	Environmental Protection Agency
	National Aeronautics and Space Administration Bioresearch; Space Medicine; Bioenvironmental Systems; Planetary Biology and Quarantine
	National Science Foundation Biological, Behavioral, and Social Sciences
	President's Council on Employment of the Handicapped
	President's Council on Physical Fitness and Sports
	Committee on Mental Retardation

United States Public Health Service

The largest federal agency for health, both in extent of influence and variety of work, is the United States Public Health Service (USPHS), headed by the Surgeon General. The United States Government Organization[11] cites as its purpose "promoting and assuring the highest level of health attainable for every individual and

Table 3-3 DHEW Components in Health Affairs

Office of Human Development
  Administration on Aging
  Office of Child Development
  Rehabilitation Services Administration
Public Health Service
  Alcohol, Drug Abuse, and Mental Health Administration
  National Institutes of Health
    Clinical Center
    Fogarty International Center
    Office of Protection from Research Risks
    National Cancer Institute
    National Heart, Lung, and Blood Institute
    National Institute for Allergy and Infectious Diseases
    National Arthritis, Metabolism, Degenerative Diseases Institute
    National Institute for Child Health and Human Development
    National Institute on Aging
    National Institute of Dental Research
    National Institute of Environmental Health Sciences
    National Institute of General Medical Sciences
    National Institute of Neurology, Communication Diseases and Stroke
    National Eye Institute
    National Institute of Mental Health
    National Institute of Alcohol Abuse and Alcoholism
    National Institute of Drug Abuse
National Library of Medicine
Division of Computer Research and Technology
Center for Disease Control
Food and Drug Administration
  Bureau of Drugs; Bureau of Foods; Bureau of Biologics; National Center for Toxicological Research; Bureau of Radiological Health; Bureau of Veterinary Medicine; Bureau of Medical Devices and Diagnostic Products
  Health Resources Administration
    Bureau of Health Planning and Resources Development
    Bureau of Health Manpower
  National Center for Health Statistics
  National Center for Health Services Research
  Health Services Administration
    Bureau of Community Health Services
    Indian Health Services Headquarters
    Bureau of Medical Services
    Bureau of Quality Assurance
Social and Rehabilitation Service
Veterans Administration

family. It is also responsible for collaborating with governments of other countries and with international organizations in world health activities." The major functions of the Service are:

1 To identify health hazards in products and services which enter one's life, to develop and promulgate, and assure compliance with, standards of control of such hazards

2 To support the development of and improve the organization, and delivery of, comprehensive and coordinated physical and mental health services for all Americans, and provide direct health care services to limited federal beneficiary populations

3 To conduct and support research in the medical and related sciences, promoting the dissemination of knowledge in these sciences and further development of health education and training to ensure an adequate supply of health manpower

Direction of the Public Health Service is a responsibility of the Assistant Secretary of Health, Education and Welfare (Health and Scientific Affairs), to whom the Surgeon General is responsible. Advisory councils are utilized to provide overall advice and policy guidance in each major program area. Regional staffs of the Public Health Service work with state authorities in developing plans, programs, and budgets for cooperative health programs.

The relationships of the USPHS to state and local governments are guided by definitions of spheres and extent of powers. Mustard[12] explains these definitions as follows:

> The federal government may assist and advise the state on its internal health affairs, but not supersede it, as the authority of each is distinct. The local government, however, has only the authority which the state delegates to it. Though the state may assume control, it seldom does. To do so would be somewhat comparable to the situation where the state militia supersedes the local sheriff or police under martial law. Of course, there are critical situations in which this may be necessary and expected.

National Institutes of Health

The National Institutes of Health (NIH), located in Bethesda, Maryland, comprise the largest single research institution in the world. A highly readable and accurate account of the history of the National Institutes of Health is available in the book by Strickland[20]. It has been appraised as "the definitive history of a phenomenon unique in the history of science—the rise to political power of biomedical research." It recounts the interacting forces of legislators, scientists, and lobbyists in the transformation of a relatively small federal microbiological laboratory into the prestigious NIH, with its many fields of action and research.

FEDERAL INFLUENCES ON HEALTH CARE DELIVERY SYSTEMS

Aside from the obvious influence of research and development such as that conducted by the NIH, federal health programs having different focuses have a marked impact on all segments of health care activities. For example, Medicare became effective in July 1966, making 19 million Americans eligible at that time for government-supported medical care in institutions approved for participation. Somers and Somers[18] have chronicled this development carefully, giving "behind the scenes" descriptions of the maneuvering and championing that went into the passage of the Medicare law, as well as the contributing forces of the health care delivery systems' interests and needs. Not only does Medicare support costs of hospitalization, etc., but it has significant influence on the quality of care through its regulations governing the eligibility of institutions for participation in the plan. Cost accounting is required, and extends to efforts to identify actual costs of education in the clinical setting, for example. This, in turn, is having effects on program planning and financing.

There are those who characterize the American apparatus as a nonsystem because of the variation of availability of care, responsiveness, and quality. However, a number of factors provide impetus for improving the system of health care delivery in the United States as well as in other countries. For example, advances in science, the rise of multi-specialty group practice, needs of special groups of people, and the cost of medical care all contribute to the climate calling for change.

The physician is in a vulnerable position in the debate about health delivery systems, and often becomes a lightning rod toward which bolts of criticism are directed. Schwartz[16] directs attention to the positive aspects of American medicine and makes some important observations, though his advocacy for the physician-defendant may be "a case of underdeveloped analysis and rhetorical overkill." Once again, one is reminded that it is not a matter of either/or, but the gray areas in between that must be dealt with effectively.

From the point of view of his experience in government, Ribicoff[6] addresses the problems of the delivery of health care in terms of the policy-making process. He admits that, although appropriate and equitable care is everyone's right, implementing the means to meet that right "is a complex and awesome task." The many entrants in the race to introduce and subsequently produce legislation have yet to provide a consensus for an acceptable, effective, and economically feasible plan. In comparing Swedish, British, and American systems, Anderson[3] provides interesting data that could be useful in the decision-making processs. Some of the advantages demonstrated by other systems will no doubt be incorporated into drafting an improved American system. The difficulty of drafting a critical part of that improved system in the form of national health insurance is demonstrated by the fact that after more than a decade of effort, no proposal put forward has found enough support even to begin the long process involved in translating a proposal into law.

Other efforts to improve the American health care system have been implemented in national legislation, most notably in Professional Standards Review Organizations (PSRO) (PL 92–603) and Health Systems Agencies (PL 93–641). PSRO is the machinery by which the quality of health care is monitored by peers. It began with physicians, and now has been extended to other health professions groups. The PSRO legislation was greeted with howls of anguish from physician groups that cited governmental interference in the so-called sacred patient/physician relationship. Since its implementation in 1974, local PSROs have developed and are functioning reasonably well enough so that the Joint Commission on-Accreditation of Hospitals now includes PSRO participation in its criteria. An example of the effect of peer review is provided by the prototype experience in New Mexico. When Medicaid costs spiraled, the state wanted to drop the program. This led physicians to form a voluntary review program. The results were reduction of overutilization and improvements when underutilization was found. Within a year, all restrictions on Medicaid benefits were lifted, and there were significant savings so that payments to doctors could be more realistic. Similar benefits of PSRO are expected to result from its use by other health professionals.

The National Health Planning and Resources Development Act of 1974 (PL 93–641) builds on the experiences of previous health resources programs such as the Hill-Burton Program, the Comprehensive Health Planning Program, Regional Medical Program, and the Experimental Health Services Delivery Systems Program. It seeks to combine their best features into one health planning and resources development effort. The Act provides for the formation of Health Systems Agencies (HSAs) and State Health Planning and Development Agencies (SHPDAs), which are to play a major role in planning, review, and approval. Each HSA is required to have a governing board with specific ratios of consumers to providers of health care, and other characteristics as follows:

> A majority (but not more than 60% of the members) shall be residents of the health service area served by the entity who are consumers of health care and who are not . . . providers of health care and who are broadly representative of the social, economic, linguistic and racial populations, geographic areas of the health service area, and major purchasers of health care. The remainder of the members shall be residents of the health service area served by the agency who are providers of health care and who represent (I) physicians (particularly practicing physicians), dentists, nurses, and other health professionals, (II) health care institutions (particularly hospitals, long-term care facilities, and health maintenance organizations), (III) health care insurers, (IV) health professional schools, and (V) the allied health professions.

The Health Systems Agencies are responsible for monitoring applications for new construction, expansion or renovation of health care facilities, and participating in systematic planning in use of scarce resources. HSAs are supported by federal funds for their operational expenses, and are therefore subject to the uncertainties common to obtaining appropriations. Progress has been slower than hoped, with 134 HSAs formed by 1976, but those that have been operational for some time report that their efforts have resulted in significant savings.

Parents' and nutritionists' use of the Federal Trade Commission's (FTC) jurisdiction in television advertising provides an interesting example of how an issue in health can be dealt with outside the usual agencies for health. The proliferation of ready-sweetened cold cereals and the fact that they are featured in TV programs for children five times as often as other cereals roused consumer activists. Two organizations joined together in the campaign—Action for Children's Television and the Center for Science in the Public Interest. Their arguments were that the prime consumers of such cereals are children; breakfast cereal is a vitamin-enriched dietary staple, unlike snacks that lay no claim to nutritional merit; sugared cereals are often eaten as snacks without milk, which makes the sugar more likely to remain on the teeth; and sweetened cereals are overpriced as well as oversugared. The FTC ruling announced in early 1978 puts restrictions on advertising for these cereals and other sugar-rich products such as candies. Manufacturers are expected to pursue an appeal of the ruling.

STATE DEPARTMENT OF HEALTH

The pattern of organization of the state health department varies from state to state, but all are broad in scope, covering many aspects of health. One of the major responsibilities of the state is promoting or assisting local (city or county) health departments. State health departments work closely with the United States Public Health Service, and are frequently the instruments through which national health programs are carried out. A major part of the state's influence is seen in its authority to grant financial aid to local health departments and to provide them with special personnel when needed. The state health department may also have some regulatory powers, such as licensing health personnel and enforcing pure food laws.

The general organizational pattern of a state health department reveals the variety of responsibilities and services involved.

LOCAL PUBLIC HEALTH ORGANIZATIONS

As with all public health organizations, the local boards of health (city or county, depending on population and need) are concerned with preserving and improving the health of the people within their

State Health Department

Commissioner of Health	
Board of Health	**Board of Supervisors**
Director, Division of Administration (including public information)	Director, Division of Public Health Nursing
Director, Division of Communicable Diseases	Director, Division of School Health Supervision
Director, Division of Laboratories and Research	Director, Division of Public Health Education
Director, Division of Chronic Diseases	Director, Division of Dental Services
Director, Division of Mental Hygiene	Director, Division of Institutions (Hospitals, Nursing Homes)
Director, Division of Maternal and Child Health	Director, Division of Sanitation
	Director, Division of Vital Statistics
Officers of Local Health Services	

boundaries. Like the state organizations, local boards of health vary somewhat in their patterns and services. Again, we may assume a typical pattern to be similar to the following:

Preventive Medicine Services The control centers for communicable diseases provide immunization programs, case-findings, and follow-up investigations to discover sources of disease. In addition, there is a heart disease control center; a venereal disease control center, offering diagnosis and treatment; and a tuberculosis control center, offering diagnostic services and follow-up care.

Administration and Special Services This category includes public health laboratories, statistics and records, budgets and accounts, and public health ordinances.

Health Centers Services These centers provide neighborhood and home services. Public health nurses work with individuals and families in homes and school centers. School health programs offer examination, immunization, and health education. Dental hygiene programs promote and protect dental health by examination and education services.

Environmental Sanitation Services These services cover a wide variety of activities. Community sanitation departments control refuse disposal, dumping areas, and accumulation of water disposal. Mosquito control programs, essential to prevent the spread of malaria and viral diseases associated with this insect vector, are handled by this department. Rat control is an important battle waged by sanitation services through eradication and refuse disposal. Restaurants and other public food purveyors are subject to inspection to guard against food contamination and to maintain standards of sanitation in food handling. Other food-related divisions enforcing regulations in specific areas are milk control and meat inspection. Health standards in pasteurization, bottling, and distribution of milk and milk-product supplies are included in a dairy division. Ordinances and other laws relating to meat products, assuring that meat is from healthy animals slaughtered in clean surroundings and prepared in a safe and sanitary process, are enforced by the sanitation services division.

Programs in public health respond like sensitive barometers to needs and problems as they arise. The need for action may be in such areas as mental health, accident prevention, and screening for metabolic disorders which lead to serious consequences for the individual and the public. Of great concern is the whole problem of water and air pollution by the usual contaminants, as well as from radioactive fallout.

VOLUNTARY HEALTH ORGANIZATIONS

America is uniquely fortunate in having an abundance of voluntary health organizations (nonprofit groups staffed in part by unsalaried, nonprofessional personnel) which contribute immeasurably to the nation's health through research, direct assistance to patients, and public education. The 1971 (seventh revision) of the *American Medical Association Directory of National Voluntary Health Organizations*[2] lists fifty such organizations. This list is incomplete, because it includes only those organizations which requested inclusion in the directory. Inclusion does not imply AMA approval, nor does absence from the list imply disapproval. AMA policy statements and guidelines are given in the introduction. The opening paragraph of the introduction to this valuable compendium of information states:

> The American voluntary health movement is a unique phenomenon which embodies three major freedoms—freedom of the individual,

freedom of enterprise, and freedom of association. National voluntary health agencies have now become an accepted part of our culture. The national voluntary health agencies offer a wealth of opportunity for dedicated citizens to freely associate to promote good health in their community, state, and country. They reflect the interest and concern of the American public with the improvement of health and eradication of disease. They are effective channels through which individuals can actively demonstrate an interest in community affairs.

The introduction then proceeds to list suggested guides for relationships between these agencies and medicine; considerations in establishing relationships between medical societies and voluntary health agencies, mutual obligations, the role of physicians, suggested medical society activities to promote understanding of voluntary health agencies, and guiding principles to relationships at the national level. Criteria for evaluation of medical programs of national agencies and recommended guidelines for relationships between voluntary health agencies and governmental health programs complete the introduction.

In some cases, it is difficult to measure the degree to which the several types of health agencies succeed in achieving their goals, and to assess their relative importance. One parameter which does provide some information is that of finances; this is revealing. The total national income of the agencies on the list which volunteered financial information amounted to $401,332,224 in 1971, while expenditures amounted to $376,650,333.

Under the heading "Health Organizations" are listed The People-to-People Health Foundation, Inc., Medic Alert Foundation International, AMA Education and Research Foundation, American National Red Cross, National Health Council, and United Health Foundations, Inc.

A wide range of primary interest, or specific disease focus, is immediately apparent from the list given below. (The number in parentheses indicates the number of units or organizations within each category.)

Alcoholism (1)	Birth defects (1)
Allergic diseases (1)	Blindness and sight (6)
Arthritis (1)	Brain (1)

Cancer (3)
Cerebral palsy (1)
Cystic fibrosis (1)
Diabetes (1)
Drug abuse (1)
Epilepsy (2)
Genetics (1)
Handicapped and crippled (1)
Hearing (1)
Hemophilia
Homemaker services (1)
Kidney (1)
Leprosy (1)

Lung diseases (1)
Maternal health (4)
Medical research (1)
Mental health (1)
Multiple sclerosis (1)
Myasthenia gravis (1)
Paraplegia (1)
Parkinson's disease (1)
Pituitary (1)
Rehabilitation (1)
Retardation (1)
Sex education (1)
Social diseases (1)

The information provided about each agency is organized under five major headings; key personnel, major purpose, organizational structure, financing and fund raising, and program (which includes research, education, and patient service). A valuable addition is a section on Continuing Education Professional Programs of Voluntary Health Agencies.

Income for these agencies is obtained by membership fees, donations and trust funds, bequests, investments, and sale of seals (e.g., American Lung Association—formerly the National Tuberculosis and Respiratory Disease Association). The value of these agencies to the American people is obvious from the support they give in terms of money and voluntary services. As is typical of the tendency for organizational self-preservation, as the major goals of an agency are realized, it frequently assumes another related goal. Examples in this area are seen in the National Foundation—March of Dimes, and the National Tuberculosis and Health Association. When founded in 1938, the March of Dimes was focused on supporting research and patient services in poliomyelitis. Now that poliomyelitis is no longer a common disease in America, the National Foundation is concerned with the causes and prevention of birth defects. A similar pattern is seen in the shift from major emphasis on tuberculosis to the more general area of lung diseases, once the scourge of tuberculosis came under control. This shift is signaled by the change in name to American Lung Association.

HOME CARE PROGRAMS

In determining how the patient's health care needs can best be met, the factors to consider are the patient's emotional and financial resources and how to make economical use of professional service, equipment, and institutions. Often both the patient and his family may feel that the home environment is more conducive to progress in recovery than the hospital. Long-term stays in the hospital are expensive. Some patients may not need daily attention from medical personnel, and, though incapacitated, may require only the help that can easily be given by the family under skilled supervision. The responsibility of providing skilled supervision has long been met by community agencies such as public health nursing.

A much more comprehensive plan of home care programs has, in recent years, developed under the aegis of the American Hospital Association (AHA). In these programs, professional and institutional services and community agencies coordinate their activities to provide higher levels of home care. Patients are admitted to these organized home care programs in much the same way they are admitted to hospitals, and thus become eligible for the services offered. As outlined by the AHA, home care programs must be able to provide the following:

Medical care and supervision
Consultant services
Nursing care and/or nursing supervision
Hospital in-patient service
Social service
Nutritional guidance
Laboratory and radiology service
Pharmaceutical service

Also included as the need dictates are physical therapy, occupational therapy, speech therapy, appliance equipment, and sterile supply service, home-delivered meal service, transportation service, and homemaker and home health-aid service. Many states include home health care agencies under their institutional licensing laws.

As shown in Table 3-4, in 1975 2,254 home health service programs were certified for Medicare reimbursement. A voluntary

**Table 3-4   Types and Numbers of
Home Health Services,
1975, Certified for Medicare
Benefits**

Type	Number
Governmental	1259
Visiting Nurse Association	530
Other voluntary agencies	47
Hospital-based	270
Miscellaneous	148
Total	2254

Source: Health Resource Statistics: Health Manpower and Health Facilities, 1975, DHEW, PHS, HRA, National Center for Health Statistics, Rockville, MD, 1975, p. 447.

accreditation program for community nursing service was begun by the National League for Nursing (NLN) and the American Public Health Association (APHA) in 1966. This has recently been broadened to include components in homemaker and home health-aide services, nutrition, occupational therapy, physical therapy, speech and hearing, and social work. The professional societies for each of these services collaborated with NLN and APHA in development of standards for accreditation that went into effect in 1976.

HEALTH MAINTENANCE ORGANIZATIONS

Various forms of prepaid health care have been provided by government and industry for 50 years. The railroad industry pioneered its implementation in the mid-nineteenth century, but it was not used until the 1920s by other groups. An interesting historical note is that a group of Texas teachers, working with Baylor Hospital in Dallas, formed a prepaid hospital insurance program that became the prototype for the Blue Cross system, which now has at least 70 member plans throughout the nation. By the 1960s, there were at least 500 "independent" programs in operation, which are not supported by major insurance organizations.

Federal authorization and funding for Health Maintenance Organization (HMO) planning and development came in 1971 as part of the revision of Medicare benefits, and the first experimental HMOs under this legislation began operation in 1972. While the benefits may vary among programs, most of them provide comprehensive care through group practice to voluntary enrollees who prepay on a capitation basis. The HMO Act of 1973 (PL 93–222) describes the components of the HMO to be available for full federal benefits as follows:

> Basic HMO care must include consultant and referral physician services, inpatient hospital services and outpatient services, hospital emergency care, home health services, diagnostic laboratory work, therapeutic radiology services, short-term outpatient mental health care, voluntary family planning services, alcohol and drug abuse services, preventive dental and eye care for children, and physical checkups, vaccinations, and health education. HMO's are additionally required to provide or arrange for specific supplemental health services such as prescription drugs, long-term physical medicine including physical therapy, and services available through intermediate and long-term care facilities.

According to the most recent information publicly available, in May 1975, there were 173 HMO-type prepaid medical care plans supported in part by federal funds, operating in 33 states, Washington, D.C., and Guam. These plans serve about 5.7 million members. Five of the plans meet all of the qualifications stipulated in the 1973 act.

REFERENCES

1 Alford, R. R., "Health Care Politics: Ideological and Interest Group Barriers to Reform," University of Chicago Press, Chicago, 1975.
2 "American Medical Association Directory of National Voluntary Health Organizations (1971)," American Medical Association, Chicago, 1971.
3 Anderson, O. W., "Health Care: Can There Be Equality?" John Wiley & Sons Inc., New York, 1972.
4 Axelrod, S. J., A. Donabedian, and D. W. Gentry (eds.), "Medical Care Chart Book," 6th ed., University of Michigan, Ann Arbor, 1976.
5 Burns, Eveline M., "Health Services for Tomorrow: Trends and Issues," Harvard University Press, Cambridge, Mass., 1973.

6 Department of Health, Education, and Welfare, Public Health Service, Health Maintenance Organizations, *Federal Register* **39** (203), Oct. 18, 1974.

7 Enos, Darryl D., "The Sociology of Health Care: Sociological, Economic, and Political Perspectives," Frederick A. Praeger Inc., New York, 1977.

8 Ginzberg, Eli, What Next in Health Policy, *Science,* **188:**1184–1186, June 20, 1975.

9 LaPatra, J. W., "Health Care Delivery Systems," Charles C Thomas Publishers, Springfield, Ill., 1975.

10 Levey, S., and N. P. Loomba, "Health Care Administration: A Managerial Perspective," J. B. Lippincott Co., Philadelphia, 1973.

11 McTaggert, A. C., and L. M. McTaggert, "Health Care Dilemma," Holbrook Press, Boston, 1976.

12 Mustard, Henry S., "An Introduction to Public Health," 3d ed., The Macmillan Company, New York, 1953, pp. 51, 52.

13 Rettig, Richard, "The Story of the National Cancer Act of 1971," Princeton University Press, Princeton, N.J., 1977.

14 Roemer, Milton I., "Health Care Systems in World Perspective," Health Administration Press, Ann Arbor, Mich., 1976.

15 Roman, Paul (ed.), "Social Perspectives on Community Mental Health," F. A. Davis Co., Philadelphia, 1974.

16 Schwartz, Harry, "The Case for American Medicine," David McKay Company, Inc., New York, 1972.

17 Seay, J. D. (ed.), "National Health Directory," J. T. Grupenhoff, Publisher, Washington, D.C., 1977.

18 Somers, H. R. and A. R. Somers, "Medicare and the Hospitals: Issues and Prospects," The Brookings Institution, Washington, D.C., 1967.

19 Somers, A. R., "Health Care in Transition: Directions for the Future," Hospital Research and Educational Trust, Chicago, 1971.

20 Strickland, S. P., "Politics, Science and Dread Disease. A Short History of United States Medical Research Policy," Harvard University Press, Cambridge, Mass., 1972.

21 Twaddle, A. C., "A Sociology of Health," The C. V. Mosby Company, St. Louis, 1977.

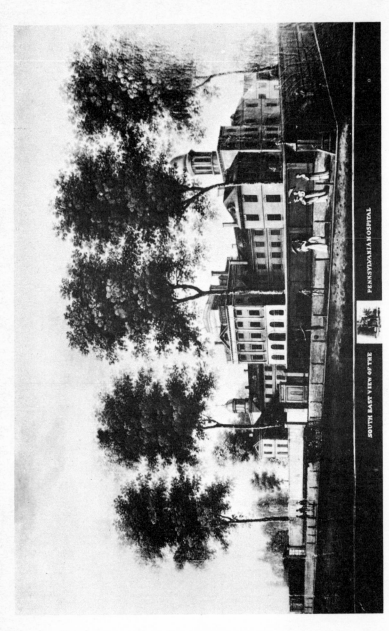

America's oldest hospital in its early days. (Courtesy of Pennsylvania Hospital, Philadelphia.)

4

HISTORY AND DEVELOPMENT OF HOSPITALS

From simple beginnings, hospitals have developed into some of the most complex institutions of society. This statement can be applied to functions, professional organization, and labor forces. A review of the forces and events that have brought them to this point is helpful in understanding the problems and opportunities of modern hospitals. The history of their development demonstrates that they have been shaped by a variety of forces active in the social order of their times, and that hospitals reflect the societal philosophy of each succeeding age.

ANCIENT AND MEDIEVAL FORERUNNERS OF THE HOSPITAL

Though crude and degrading to those whose disease brought them there, the leper colonies may be thought of as the first "hospitals." One must put the term in quotation marks because they were not serving a function aimed at helping the individual, but of protecting society from them. For example, for centuries the leper was a symbol of contagion, and set apart from society by custom and law. In western civilization, providing places for the sick began to develop in the first centuries AD, though much of the concern was motivated by self-serving aims.

Any aid given the poor by the early hospitals was in fact a device directed toward securing grace and salvation, reflecting the teaching of St. Chrystosom (344–407) that "the poor are healers of your wounds." As Rosen[10] indicates, "They were not primarily concerned with medical care, but spiritual issues." With the influx of pilgrims journeying to Rome came the establishment of wayside shelters called hospices, and from hospice comes the derivation of the hospital in name as well as in function, for frequently enough, those in need of shelter were ill.

The Crusades were another impetus to the development of hospitals, for the wounded and sick crusaders needed care that, in their homelands, would have been provided by the family. These hospitals were staffed in part by women, and physicians and surgeons were assigned to direct them. The monastic orders of the medieval church were instrumental in establishing charitable houses and hospitals. The general pattern was of a centrally located infirmary or almshouse, hostels for pilgrims near the city gates, and leper houses outside the gates. The medieval hospital system may have been motivated by the need to care for the sick poor, but it also served to clear the streets of repugnant sights.

RENAISSANCE AND REFORMATION

In England, the hospital system crumbled and disappeared along with the dissolution of monasteries between 1536 and 1539, having reached a peak of 245 hospitals in the fourteenth century. Lacking church sponsorship, those hospitals remaining were put under civic authority, and were used to house the incurably ill and homeless. The Reformation made less of an impact outside England because elsewhere the monastic hospitals were readily placed under state control.

ENLIGHTENMENT

The new humanitarian spirit of the eighteenth and early nineteenth centuries had its effect on facilities for serving the sick. In England, for example, 154 new hospitals were supported by interested subscribers who volunteered their money and their efforts. The hospital became a place dedicated to the "relief and maintenance of curable poor people." The significant difference here is the change from "incurable" to "curable." The first hospitals established in the United States were the Pennsylvania Hospital in Philadelphia (1751) and New York Hospital (1773).

LATE NINETEENTH AND EARLY TWENTIETH CENTURIES

Until the development of the basic sciences, most particularly bacteriology and human physiology, hospitals remained charitable institutions working on an empirical basis. With the gradual shift toward scientific medicine that began in the middle of the nineteenth century, the hospitals began to utilize medical and surgical intervention, thus making great advances in the care of the sick by adding the dimension of treatment. Anesthesia and listerian antisepsis were introduced into surgery, and further scientific investigation and integration of findings into medicine. The merging of science with humanitarian motivation has brought us to our modern concepts of health care, and is a major factor influencing the course health care is to take in the future.

THE HOSPITAL AND THE MEDICAL PROFESSION

Any review of the history of hospitals must also take into account the medical profession, the people themselves. In the sixteenth and seventeenth centuries, the "medical profession" included the town leech, the compassionate monk caring for his charges, and the charlatan friar pretending miraculous cures. Science in medicine came with the Renaissance, when the natural scientist began to see and think for himself.

Organization of the medical profession came about independently of hospitals, the most notable such organization being the Royal College of Physicians, established by Henry VIII in England in 1518. However, there were several bonds which kept the physician in close association with hospitals: his humanitarian response evoked by firsthand knowledge of suffering; his appetite for increased knowledge and experience in the causes and cures of disease; and his responsibility as a teacher to share his knowledge and experience with those qualified to continue the growth of medical science.

By the nineteenth century, physicians found the hospital to be essential for the care of major illness. From his partisan view, the physician began to think of the hospital less as an agency of society, and more as "his" hospital.

Nursing, though as old as motherhood, became a profession in medicine through the efforts of Florence Nightingale, who established the first school of nursing after the Crimean War, in 1856. This school was not, however, a part of a hospital. Thirty years later, hospital schools of nursing were established in America, and nursing became a profession associated with hospital care of the sick. Although nursing has branched out to cover wider areas, the fundamental education is in the hospital milieu.

Broadening concepts of patient care have led to the development of a number of new (within the last fifty years) professions in the health field. Concomitantly, there has also been the development of services for those who are not necessarily ill but are incapacitated in some way, and thus do not fit the general definition, patient. They may be termed clients.

Public health services also contribute to health in ways other than direct patient care. More will be said about these services in a subsequent chapter, but it is significant to remember that these health services for the most part had their beginnings in, and still are active in, hospitals, both in service and education. Still another area of rapidly developing health service occupations encompasses the various technologies.

THE HOSPITAL AND CONTEMPORARY SOCIETY

Today, there is no such thing as *the* hospital; there are hospitals. Among them, there are more differences than similarities in their programs, sizes, aims, resources, and histories.

Hospital goals have gradually shifted over the years in response to changes in philosophy, scientific knowledge, and perceptions of the varied services possible. It is possible to speak of "the hospital" of 1860, and to picture accurately an institution primarily concerned with charitable care of the needy. Today, we have to modify "hospital" in order to know just what is meant, for shifts in goals have brought about specialization. There are general hospitals for care of acute illness, short-term in scope; chronic disease hospitals involving long-term care; hospitals for specific illnesses; small community hospitals; large medical centers; government hospitals; voluntary nonprofit hospitals and the current development of academic health science centers. Each has its own characteristics. In a broad sense, the hospital is a public utility whose purpose is to serve the entire community, the well and the sick. Service to the patient is not the hospital's only role but one of a complex of services comprising education, research, and preventive and rehabilitative medicine as well.

Because the hospital is now the nerve center of medical care and all that goes into that complex, there is, inevitably, an interaction between all of the forces molding the hospital and those who work within it. As a rule, the more useful and vital a service becomes in the social order, the more certain it is to come under the influence of the functions of government. This is evident in the need for a broad base of public funds needed to protect the public from unqualified or charlatan purveyors of the service, and the increasing expense of maintaining facilities for service.

THE EVOLVING HOSPITAL CONCEPT

The varied and complex influences on health care, as well as the predicted needs of society, make planning for the future vital. Such planning efforts are demonstrated in the formation and functions of the Health Services Agencies described in Chapter 3. The importance of hospitals to society rests on three basic functions: care of the patient, extension of knowledge regarding the management and prevention of disease, and the education of health personnel. The ferment in medicine—reflected in the literature in reports of selective and comprehensive studies of the problems involved—is directly attributable to the changing needs, expectations, and value systems of society. One of the prominent studies frequently quoted is that of the Association of American Medical Colleges under the chairmanship of Dr. Lowell T. Coggeshall.[3] The Coggeshall Report identifies major trends related to health care, listing the following as "Emerging Trends":

Scientific advance
Population change

Increasing individual health expectations
Increasing effective demand for health care
Increasing specialization in medical practice
Increasing use of technological advances and equipment
Increasing use of a team approach to health care
Need for increasing numbers of physicians
Need for increasing numbers of health personnel
Expanding role of government
Rising costs

These trends are identified and discussed by other investigators, as in the Coggeshall Report, in the context of the particular purpose of their studies. One of the most readable and thought-provoking of such books in the literature on health care is Dr. Richard M. Magraw's *Ferment in Medicine*.[8] Hospitals are vitally concerned with all phases of these studies, for they constitute the major arena where the vying forces play their roles in what may become a game of life and death.

Halderman[5] warns that "making long-range predictions is a precarious business," but takes the leap from his understanding of trends in health care. Beginning with the question of what the patient of the future will be like, and what the needs will be Halderman says:

> Greater emphasis will be on early diagnosis and health maintenance. There will be more preventive rehabilitation and health education activities and less definitive treatment. In short, the hospital will become a medical health service center, strongly oriented to providing the various levels of care needed by patients with chronic illness . . . As a result of the changes in the hospital program, the percentage of the hospital's floor space devoted to the traditional nursing unit may be cut in half.

Some of Halderman's predictions are beginning to develop through the academic health sciences center concept put forward by the *Carnegie Commission Report on Higher Education and the Nation's Health*,[6] and in other respects as a response to changing needs and resources.

AREA HEALTH EDUCATION CENTERS

In 1972, the Health Resources Administration of the Bureau of Health Manpower Education, (DHEW) launched a program authorized by the Comprehensive Health Manpower Training Act of 1970 to educate health professions personnel at locations where health needs are greatest. The Area Health Education Center (AHEC) is basically a system or arrangement that links health service organizations and educational institutions in a way that serves both the communities and the students. The program is targeted on providing extended learning-experience opportunities and added health capabilities to underserved areas. Particular emphasis is to be on increasing the availability of primary care. The AHECs cooperate with hospitals and community agencies in planning and developing effective health care delivery systems, and assist in developing educational programs to meet area health personnel needs. The educational activities conducted under the guidance of the contracting university medical center include:

Clinical instruction for undergraduate health professions students

Residency training, especially in primary care specialties

Continuing education for health professions practitioners

Assistance in the development of additional educational programs for health personnel

Eleven university medical centers* from among the 25 applicants were awarded 5-year AHEC contracts in 1972. Each of the institutions addressed areas of need that were specific to its own missions and service spheres within the criteria for awarding contracts. Outreach was, and is continuing to be, the primary characteristic of each of the individual projects. With the five years of experience, evaluation of the impact and products of the eleven projects is now in progress. In 1977 two additional years of funding were authorized, and several new contracts were approved. Two of the basic premises being tested are that (1) extending the sphere of

*Universities of California at San Francisco, Illinois, Minnesota, Missouri, New Mexico, North Carolina, North Dakota, Southern California, Texas Medical Branch at Galveston, West Virginia, and Tufts University.

academic medicine to underserved areas will improve the quality of care, and that (2) students who have at least part of their professional education in these areas will find them attractive, and thus will elect to enter practice there after graduation. This aspect of comprehensive health personnel training constitutes a pilot project that translates the conceptual to the operational, and provides the means to assess the potential for large-scale implementation.

Not all types of hospitals are involved in educational programs and research. However, those that are provide essential clinical practice for many of the health professions personnel. Formal education programs conducted in hospitals include medical residencies and internships, and basic professional preparation in nursing and the allied health professions. A great deal of in-service education is given in hospitals, particularly in training supportive personnel in the many departments that make up the complete spectrum of services offered. By its very nature, clinical research involves the hospital setting, where the contributions to the expansion and dissemination of knowledge are significant in terms of benefits within the institution and in the world at large.

REFERENCES

1 Bettman, O. L., "A Pictorial History of Medicine," Charles C Thomas, Publisher, Springfield, Ill., 1962.

2 Brown, R. E., Medical Care: Its Social and Organizational Aspects, *New Eng. J. Med.*, **269:**609, 1963.

3 Coggeshall, Lowell T., "Planning for Medical Progress through Education," report to the Association of American Medical Colleges, Evanston, Ill., 1965.

4 Ellis, J. R., Medical Care: Its Social and Organizational Aspects: The Regionalization of Hospital Services, *New Eng. J. Med.*, **269:**953, 1963.

5 Halderman, J. C., The Hospital of the Future, *Public Health News*, **47:**127–131, June 1966. Publication of the New Jersey State Department of Health, Trenton, N.J.

6 "Higher Education and the Nation's Health: A Report of the Carnegie Commission," McGraw-Hill Book Company, New York,1971.

7 Jaco, E. G., Medical Care, Its Social and Organizational Aspects: Twentieth Century Attitudes toward Health and Their Effect on Medicine, *New Eng. J. Med.*, **269:**18, 1963.

8 Magraw, Richard, "Ferment in Medicine: A Study of the Essence of Medical Practice and of Its New Dimensions," W. B. Saunders Company, Philadelphia, 1966.

9 Roemer, Milton I., "Health Care Systems in World Perspective," Hospital Administration Press, Ann Arbor, Mich., 1977.

10 Rosen, G., "The Hospital: Historical Sociology of a Community Institution," Macmillan & Co., Ltd., London, 1963.

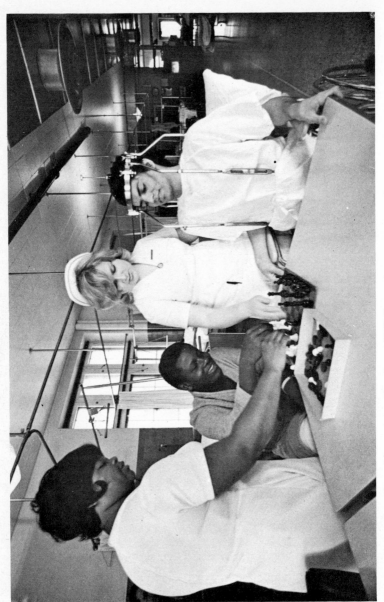

The hospital works with and for people. (*Courtesy of Bill Rogers.*)

5

SOCIOLOGIC ASPECTS OF
THE HOSPITAL

SOCIAL STRUCTURE

A hospital is a society within itself, as well as an instrument of
society at large. It is a cooperative system made up of individuals
interacting as a whole toward external elements, and as units or
group members to internal elements. The structure of this system is
the result of the reciprocal influences of the formal and informal
aspects of organization.

STRATIFICATION

Even a cursory acquaintance with a hospital society provides evidence of a highly stratified social organization. The caste system is
a way of life to all who work in a hospital. This is seen in the very
clothes worn; uniforms are everywhere apparent, and to each is
attached a symbolic or real identifying tag of status. The color of a
uniform may be that identifying tag, and most people recognize

and react to what that tag signifies. For example, when the medical technologists in one hospital were told to wear yellow uniforms rather than white there was an immediate and vociferous reaction because yellow uniforms were also worn by workers in the housekeeping department. According to the value system of the medical technologists, yellow uniforms would have been effective in downgrading them in many respects; for example, they would no longer have entree to the staff cafeteria, for no one in a yellow uniform frequented this "inner sanctum."*

Stratification is the product of power differences (influence and decision making), social distance (degree of closeness and informality), and prestige distinction (general emphasis on symbolic rank). It is a functionally related phenomenon, encouraged as a means of achieving the goals to which the hospital is committed. It is also one solution to the complexity of authoritarian chains of command. There are, in most general hospitals, two distinct lines of authority, lines which produce conflict when they cross.

The hierarchy within the hospital is based not only on social stratification but on legal responsibilities as well. The hospital's legal responsibilities are imposed by the larger social units of which hospitals and their personnel are instruments.

The importance of the physicians in the hierarchy of health agencies also signifies their unique responsibilities. As the persons licensed to practice medicine, they have a powerful voice in the management of the hospital. They are the focal point of responsibility—often in the awesome position of making life and death decisions. Although physicians, like patients, are "guests" of the hospital (unless, of course, they are salaried), they earn their high rank. It is the hospital that depends on the physician for its reason to exist: service to patients. The physicians' active participation in management is, therefore, needed and sought.

In those hospitals supporting residency and internship programs of education, the process of enculturation of the independent physician is part of informal (in the sense that there is no fixed program) socialization into the profession. The residents and in-

---

*It is not the writer's intention to downgrade the vital importance of the housekeeping personnel. Obviously, this is an important group, contributing to the well-being of everyone—patient and employee alike.

terns observe their superiors and attempt to simulate their behavior, thus perpetuating the physician image.

Among the other health services personnel employed by the hospital, there is some jostling for position and status. Nursing is generally accorded professional status, again, in part because of licensure. (However, those who give nursing care but are not professional find themselves on the lower rungs of the status ladder.) Other professions in the health field now look more and more to licensure as both a criterion and a means of attaining status. The fact remains, however, that status is as often conferred by those in the higher echelons of structure as it is earned by education and performance. Until physicians can see that their status is not threatened but is more often enhanced by acknowledging others in the health services, the battle will go on.

EFFECTS OF STRATIFICATION

One of the most pronounced effects of stratification occurs in the flow of communications. There are numerous communication blocks and diversions, particularly from lower to higher levels. Since information must be relayed from one level to the next without bypassing any, the message can be distorted in passing through "filters" of interpretation and emphasis.

Multiple subordination leads to decreased authority and the development of dependency which effectively short-circuits individual responsibility and initiative. An example of this is given by Brown[5] in her account of a mundane incident on a ward. The charge nurse had difficulty in getting the laundry room to deliver needed supplies. When the nurse had to explain why a certain patient had not been cared for as expected, the shortage of linens was one critical point. The patient's physician then called for the supplies and got them. The nurse may have been grateful to the physician, but whether this was the case or not, the nurse was also dependent on the physician for solving a problem that should have been resolved at a lower hierarchic level.

Motivation to do well in one's work can be affected by stratification. It is easy to say, "That's not part of my work," or to blame the next higher person for poor performance. The low one on the totem pole tends to feel that the work is not important and consequently performs at a minimal level. Stratification also causes fragmentation, and as a consequence the highly touted team concept falls far short of winning.

Stratification of personnel can result in conflict or, at least, in a lowering of proper self-esteem. Within the overall structure of any organization, subgroups align themselves for mutual protection in the social milieu, and for social intercourse. These may be cliques within certain larger groups, or a form of professional clannishness. So simple a thing as a coffee break can demonstrate this. Looking over the people in the coffee shop, one can see operating room nurses together, medical unit nurses together, clinical laboratory personnel together, and so on for as many different services as may be represented. Each tends to stay within its own narrow boundaries, refusing the stimulus of other points of view. Group cohesiveness shuts out "interlopers" unless they make a conscious effort to introduce themselves.

That groups impose discipline upon those who wish to remain "in" is well known. The restrictions can as easily extend to work norms as to social norms. Frequently, group members may be ostracized by their peers if they are more productive than their norms require, or even if they are more cheerful about carrying out their assignments. The accepted limitations of group behavior illumine the countless opportunities for improving group dynamics.

Patient Perception of Stratification

Status and the effects of stratification on hospital personnel are not lost on patients, particularly those who stay in the hospital long enough to discern the nuances involved. They may make use of the "system" for their own purposes to meet subconscious or recognized needs. Patients, too, tend to make group alignments. They do this for various reasons, some of which fall into the category of mutual instruction. Patients teach one another how to deal with physicians and how to keep up appearances before physicians; they compare notes on their progress and on different physicians' approaches to the same illness; and they discuss and analyze the staff members. In turn, the staff can make positive use of patient organization to assist in achieving goals for the individual members of such groups.

CLASSIFICATION OF PATIENTS

The first "sorting" process involves admission per se. If the hospital's function is to treat only specified types of diseases, or specific socioeconomic groups, those not meeting the criteria are not admitted. If the hospital is a large teaching institution, the patients may be screened for their diseases or medical problems and the admissions may be made largely on the basis of the patients' being "adequate clinical material."

The second sorting occurs at the admitting office, where patients are assigned to wards or private rooms and to nursing units organized around medical or surgical specialties. The assignments depend on the seriousness of the patient's condition, and on age and sex.

A third sorting begins as the staff of the patients' nursing unit classify them as "good" (this usually means compliant, quiet, causing no disturbance) or "bad." The more subtle classifications develop with interaction between the patients and those who care for them, reflected in people's feelings for one another, and in the meshing of opportunities to satisfy individual psychological needs.

If status is evidenced by uniforms, the patients can be lowly indeed. The ubiquitous hospital gown with its purely functional design strips the patients of any semblance of identification by clothing. Literally denuded of dignity, they are then accessible for the most probing investigation by staff and physicians. It is a great day for patients when they may once more choose and wear their own clothes, even so simple a thing as pajamas.

Side Effects of Classification

Unquestionably, important psychological and physical effects stem from the various processes of classification. It is not enough to tell patients, "You can't judge one case by another," in an effort to separate their problems from those that seem similar. Some psychic trauma is almost inevitable for the new arrival in a surgical ward housing patients in the various stages of recovery from an operation similar to the one that the new arrival is to have. The very worst fears may be confirmed—though without justification—as he or she looks over these roommates, sees what is done for and to them, and hears them talk about the operation.

Another possibility of psychic trauma that calls for the greatest understanding is occasioned by the isolation necessitated by certain types of infection. All the ramifications of isolation add up to a heavy burden for sensitive patients. They are extremely uncomfortable, and may even be pathetic in their distress at having become "a menace to society" because of the microorganisms they harbor. All of the primitive reactions to the sick role may surface, perhaps with little effect, but in some instances as an explosive mixture of feelings.

CONCLUSION

The hierarchic structure of hospitals developed gradually as a means of organizing and mobilizing the available internal resources that would achieve the hospital's goal of providing health care. Modifications of the system are needed, and as research continues and its findings are incorporated into the decisions of the authorities responsible for providing optimal health care, the necessary changes will be made. The critical element is time. The need for change may be now—or yesterday—but attitudes are long in the making, slow in the unmaking. Pressures for change will come from forces external to the hospital and, if properly directed, can be beneficial.

REFERENCES

1　Abdellah, Faye G., and Eugene Levine, "Effect of Nurse Staffing on Satisfaction with Nursing Care," American Hospital Association, Monograph Series #4, Chicago, 1958.

2　Argyris, Chris, "Diagnosing Human Relations in Organizations: A Case Study of a Hospital," Labor and Management Center, Yale University, New Haven, Conn., 1956.

3　Argyris, Chris, "Personality and Organization: The Conflict Between System and Individual," Harper & Row, Publishers, Incorporated, New York, 1957.

4 Brown, Esther Lucile, "Newer Dimensions of Patient Care: The Use of the Physical and Social Environment of the General Hospital for Therapeutic Purposes," Russell Sage Foundation, New York, 1961.

5 Brown, Esther Lucile, "Newer Dimensions of Patient Care: Improving Staff Motivation and Competence in the General Hospital," Russell Sage Foundation, New York, 1962.

6 Enos, Darryl D., "The Sociology of Health Care: Sociological, Economic, and Political Perspectives," Frederick A. Praeger Inc., New York, 1977.

7 Georgopoulos, B. S., and F. C. Mann, "The Community General Hospital," The Macmillan Company, New York, 1962.

8 Heydebrand, W. V., "Hospital Bureaucracy," Dunellen Publishing Co., Inc. New York, 1973.

9 Rakich, J. S., "Hospital Organization and Management," Catholic Hospital Association, St. Louis, 1972.

10 Roman, Paul (ed.), "Social Perspectives on Community Mental Health," F. A. Davis Company, Philadelphia, 1974.

11 Strauss, George, and J. R. Sayles, "Personnel: The Human Problems of Management," Prentice-Hall, Inc., Englewood Cliffs, N.J., 1960.

12 Twaddle, A. C., "A Sociology of Health," The C. V. Mosby Company, St. Louis, 1977.

13 Wilson, Robert N., The Primary Group in the Hospital, *Hosp. Admin.*, 3:13–23, Summer 1958.

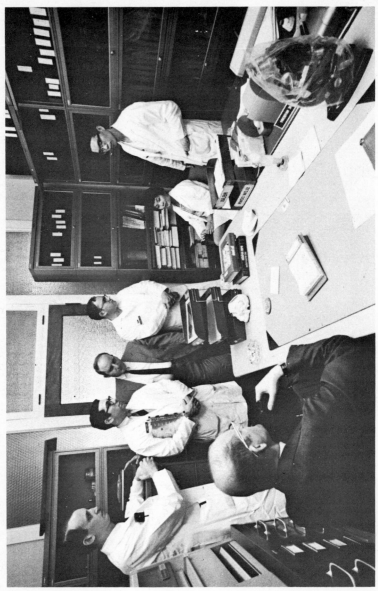

A chief of service briefs the staff. (Courtesy of Bill Pearson.)

6

ORGANIZATIONAL STRUCTURE OF HOSPITALS

Hospitals have been dubbed "a city within a city," having as they do restaurants, hotel services, laundry, library, pharmacy, educational services, and a power plant. The hospital administrator may be compared to the mayor of a city. The population of this "city" has the average educational level of a college graduate (in contrast to an average city, where the average is at the high school-junior level). The hospital is, in these details, like its personnel organizational aspects, a society.

Perrow[12] has identified four goals of a complex organization: (1) to secure inputs in the form of capital sufficient to establish itself, operate, and expand as need arises; (2) to secure acceptance in the form of basic legitimization of activity; (3) to marshal necessary skills; and (4) to coordinate the activities of its members and the relations of the organization with other organizations, and with clients or customers.

In the typical voluntary nonprofit hospital, it is the board of trustees that is primarily concerned with the first and second goals, the medical staff and administrator with the third, and the administrator with the fourth. Having a board of trustees ensures that the nonprofit status of the hospital is maintained, that funds are not misused, and that community needs are met. The medical staff advises the board of trustees as well as the administrators and also participates in major decisions based on technical knowledge the board is not expected to have. The administrator is the agent of the board; his or her job is to see that the stated goals of the institution are achieved. It is the administrator around whom all of the hospital's organizational activities converge. This person must be an expert in human relations, economics, mechanics, materials, and decision making.

CLASSIFICATION OF HOSPITALS

Two major classifications are made: (1) source of financial support or ownership, and (2) function (i.e., the type of patient and/or disease cared for). Tax-supported hospitals may be federal (USPHS or Veterans Administration hospitals), state, county, or city. Proprietary hospitals are owned by an individual or by stockholders. Voluntary nonprofit hospitals depend upon contributions, endowments, etc., in addition to patient fees, to maintain solvency.

Classifying hospitals by function reveals a wide variety ranging from the general short-term and the long-term chronic disease, to those treating a single disease or several related diseases. There are numerous hospitals for patients of specified groups, such as labor unions and industries.

ACCREDITATION OF HOSPITALS

In 1911, the American College of Surgeons made recommendations for standardizing hospitals, and in 1915, the American Hospital Association joined ACS in promoting the recommendations in a formal program and instituted an inspection system. By 1948, these two groups were joined by the American College of Physicians, the Canadian Medical Association, and the American Medical Association to form the Joint Commission on Accreditation of Hospitals

Table 6-1   Number of Hospitals: 1970 and 1975

Type of hospital	Number, 1970	Number, 1975
Total U.S.	**7,123**	**7,156**
Federal	408	382
Nonfederal	6,715	6,774
Psychiatric	519	544
Tuberculosis	101	36
Long-term general	236	215
Short-term general	5,859	5,979
Bed size		
6–24	397	299
25–49	1,327	1,155
50–99	1,490	1,481
100–199	1,275	1,363
200–299	592	678
300–399	356	378
400–499	190	230
500 and over	232	291

Source: *Hospital Statistics*, American Hospital Association, Chicago, 1976:18.

(JCAH). The commission is composed of members appointed by each of the participating organizations. The standards set by the commission are used to measure hospital efficiency and professional performance.

Accreditation review mechanisms have moved toward utilization of the hospital's own check systems in maintaining quality performance. This is consistent with the philosophy of peer review and has the further advantage of stimulating ongoing internal review and supporting good management practices. External review by JCAH then becomes a verification process, with accreditation the means of public affirmation of the quality of the institution. The JCAH publishes a monthly *Quality Review Bulletin* which features articles and current information on the subject, as well as information on JCAH standards. The quality assurance audit is a major instrument for review of performance. Criteria are established locally which are then used for monitoring performance, using the patients' records for the data base. A sample audit sheet is given in Figure 6-1. Note that the emphasis in the criteria is on

1 Audit Criteria — Audit Topic: Respiratory Therapy for Chronic Obstuctive Lung Disease

	CRIT. NO.	Elements	STANDARD 100%	STANDARD 0%	Exceptions	Instructions and Definitions for Data Retrieval
Justification		DIAGNOSIS				
	1.	Abnormal pulmonary function test (PFT) and symptoms	√		1A. None	1. Abnormal PFT = report of airway obstruction and/or hyperinflation. Symptoms = age history for dyspnea, cough, or expectoration. .
		SURGERY/SPECIAL DIAGNOSTIC OR THERAPEUTIC PROCEDURES				
	2.	Volume-cycled ventilation		√	2A. Failure of low-flow oxygen therapy	2. Volume-cycled ventilation = intubation and ventilation with MA-1 or other volume-cycled ventilator. 2A. Low-flow oxygen therapy = oxygen administered by cannula or Venturi mask. Look for flow rate of oxygen concentration. Failure of low-flow oxygen therapy = 15 mm Hg increase in pCO_2, 0.1 fall in pH, or progressive loss of consciousness.
		ADMISSION				
	3.	Impending respiratory failure; or	√		3A. None	3. Impending respiratory failure = $pCO_2 > 50$ mm Hg, $p0_2 < 60$ mm Hg, or Ph < 7.2. See arterial blood gas report.
	4.	Progressive symptoms despite outpatient therapy	√		4A. None	4. Progressive symptoms= increased dyspnea, cough, expectoration. Outpatient therapy = bronchodilators, expectorants, inhalation therapy.
Outcome		DISCHARGE STATUS				
	5.	Improved arterial blood gases	√		5A. None	5. See arterial blood gas report for 5 mm Hg decrease in pCO_2 and 5 mm Hg increase in $p0_2$ over value on admission; pH nearer 7.4.
	6.	Symptoms improved	√		6A. None	6. Dyspnea, cough, expectoration less than on admission. See MD's progress notes.
	7.	Outpatient therapy arranged			7A. None	7. Appointment made for inhalation therapy or low-flow oxygen therapy at home, MD's office, or clinic or arrangements made for medical observation.
	8.	MORTALITY		√	8A. None	
Indicators		LENGTH OF STAY				
	9.	4 to 14 days	√		9A. Patients had heart failure or pneumonia	
		OTHER				
	10.	Diagnostic admission		√	10A. Patient had impending respiratory failure or progressive symptoms despite outpatient therapy	10. Diagnostic admission = face sheet reads "patient admitted for diagnostic studies.
	11.	Readmission for respiratory failure within 1 year		√	11A. Patient admitted for treatment of disease other than COLD	
		COMPLICATIONS			CRITICAL PREVENTIVE AND RESPONSIVE MANAGEMENT	
	12.	Nosocomial infection		√	12A. Inhalation therapy equipment changed every 24 hours; or disposable or gas-sterilized nondisposable equipment used	12. Nosocomial infection = sputum or blood culture report of organism not present on original culture, temperature > 37.8 C (100 F), and leukocytosis.
	13.	Tracheal stenosis in patient previously intubated		√	13A. Tube removed or replaced via tracheostomy after 72 hours; and 13B. Cuff deflated every hour.	13. Look for complication in records of patients readmitted after intubation.

Figure 6-1 Suggested criteria for an audit of respiratory therapy for chronic obstructive lung disease (COLD). *(Source: W. B. Buckingham: "COLD War: Rationale for Criteria to Assess Respiratory Therapy,"* Quality Review Bulletin, *September 1977, p. 23. Reprinted with permission. Note: Publication does not infer official approval by*

their being understandable, written in behavioral terms, measurable, and achievable.

JCAH accreditation site visits are made by a team with expertise in assessing compliance with the standards. The team conducts interviews with key persons, reviews patient-care audit documents, departmental records, and minutes of hospital committees, and visits as many services and departments as are indicated. The site visit also includes an assessment of the physical plant of the institution. The team prepares a report that includes identification of standards in which there is noncompliance, recommendations for improvement, and commendations as indicated. The team weighs all the evidence in making its recommendation to the Commission. The options are:

> Full accreditation for three years (new or renewal)
> Probationary accreditation (usually for one year)
> Withholding accreditation from a new applicant
> Revoking accreditation previously granted

JCAH accreditation is important, not only in terms of the public affirmation it carries, but as one of the conditions by which hospitals qualify for grants, participation in the Medicare program, and specialized accreditation of educational programs offered.

BASIC ORGANIZATION

Over the many years in which hospitals have been developing, what might have appeared to be haphazard organization was actually formed in response to the individual needs of the individual institutions, their problems and services. The principal influences on the evolution of organizational patterns have been, and are yet, concern for quality care and efficient business operation. A typical chart of organizational structure for hospitals is shown in Figure 6-2.

Major divisions of organization are business and finance, physical plant, laundry, nursing, dietary and food service, other professional services, and education. In some instances, research will be found as one of these divisions, but as a rule research activities are a part of one of the basic divisions. Education includes that for basic professional qualification, continuing education, and in-service education. Nursing service is the largest division because

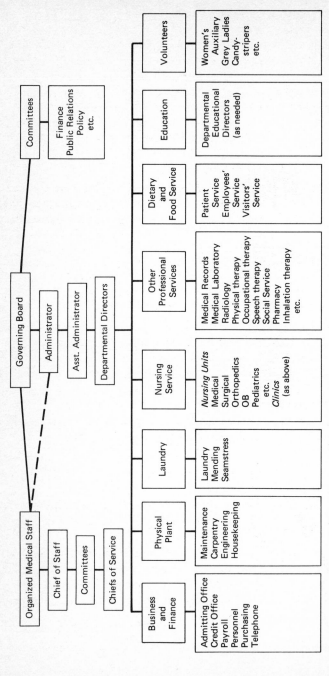

Figure 6-2 Chart of typical hospital staff organization.

daily round-the-clock staffing is required, whereas the responsibilities of the other divisions are time-limited, though available after regular hours on an emergency-call basis. Radiology and clinical laboratory services may be maintained for day and evening shifts, and on-call for the night hours.

Institutional Administrative Organization

The governing board of a hospital is generally made up of persons representing a variety of professional and business groups who are interested in community needs and services. They serve as volunteers in that they are nonsalaried. (The exception is the profit-oriented proprietary hospital, whose board members are often stockholders.) Board members with various backgrounds are valuable assets in meeting the many problems that attend hospital operations. The board has the ultimate legal responsibility for the hospital's activities outside of actual medical practice. The medical staff works closely with the board but is not completely subordinate to the board, as is the administrator.

The hospital administrator is the agent of the governing board, implementing its stated policies, and advising the board in the formulation of policies. In large institutions he or she may have a staff of administrative assistants, each of whom is responsible for a given division or combination of divisions. The division (or departmental) supervisors are next in the line of authority, each an expert in his own area. Under the division supervisors are the subsection supervisors who are responsible for the work of staff members.

The hospital is an organization concerned with (1) selection, (2) supply, of things and people, (3) service, (4) communication, (5) environmental control, (6) discovery through research, and (7) education. Its complexity is bound to produce problems, and these are, in great measure, the daily work of administration, both institutional and medical.

Medical Staff Organization

The medical staff of a hospital is a select group of physicians and dentists who, by their membership, are granted the privilege of using the hospital's facilities for their patients. The medical staff has its own pattern of organization which, in some respects, parallels that of the institutional organization. It constitutes a second (but not subordinate) structure of authority. Balancing two separate but equal lines of authority is, of itself, a source of some knotty problems, some of which are keenly felt in the lower echelons of the organization. Smith[14] has reviewed this dilemma of the hospital, and Brown[4] has a great deal to say about it in her monographs on patient care.

In Figure 6-2, the position of the medical staff organization is only briefly indicated. Note that the line relationships between the medical staff and the hospital administrator are reciprocally advisory. A variety of committees, ranging from the credentials committee to the infection committee, implement the purposes of the medical staff to assure quality patient care. The medical staff is organized along parliamentary lines, with elected officers, executive committee ("cabinet"), and special appointive committees. It generally meets once a month.

One of the most powerful committees is the credentials committee, which investigates applicants for admission to the medical staff membership, making sure that the applicant is qualified by education, training, and experience to practice medicine using the hospital's facilities. The results of this investigation are reported to the executive committee, which then recommends appointment of staff members to the governing board. The governing board is legally responsible for making these appointments.

Medical specialty boards may define the qualifications for eligibility for staff privileges. An example of such a statement is given in the following description approved by the Regents of the American College of Surgeons in June 1976.

Statement on Qualifications for Surgical Privileges in Approved Hospitals*
I Qualifications of the responsible surgeon

> *Eligibility to perform hospital surgical procedures as the responsible surgeon must be based on an individual's education, training, experience, and demonstrated proficiency.*

A Acceptable education will consist of graduation from a medical school approved by the Council on Medical Education of the American Medical Association, or from a foreign school acceptable

*Bulletin of the American College of Surgeons, April 1977. Reprinted with permission.

to the medical licensing board of the state, plus education leading to qualification as a surgical specialist.

B A "surgical specialist" is defined as a physician who:

Is certified by an American surgical specialty board approved by the American Board of Medical Specialties; or

By reason of his education, training, and experience, has been judged eligible by such a board for its examination; or

Is a Fellow of the American College of Surgeons; or

Has obtained, in a country outside the United States, graduate surgical education which satisfies the training requirements for Fellowship in the American College of Surgeons.

It is recognized that surgical procedures may also be performed by physicians who do not meet this definition, under the following conditions:

1 A physician who received the MD degree prior to 1968 and who has had full surgical privileges for over five years in a hospital approved by the Joint Commission on Accreditation of Hospitals where most of his surgical practice is conducted; or

2 A physician who renders surgical care in (a) an emergency, or (b) an area of limited population where a surgical specialist is not available; or

3 A physician who has just finished formal training in an approved surgical residency program as defined in his specialty, for whom the appropriate surgical board has not yet determined eligibility.

C The granting and continuation of surgical privileges will be based upon the staff member's record of demonstrated performance as evaluated by an established hospital peer review mechanism and medical audit. Requests for privileges not generally associated with the field in which the applicant has been trained must be specifically requested and documented with evidence of appropriate training and experience.

In certain geographically isolated and sparsely settled areas, fully trained surgeons in various fields may not be available. The performance of certain surgical procedures, especially of an emergency nature, by a physician without special surgical training may be in the best interest of the public in that area. The medical staff and the governing body of hospitals in such areas should periodically review the quality, the number, and the variety of surgical procedures being performed, as well as the surgical referral policies of the staff. It is possible that the referral pattern in surgical care is such as to discourage the application of properly trained and qualified surgeons for staff membership.

II. Qualifications of surgical assistants in the operating room

In the absence of specifically trained and readily available surgical operating room assistants for a great number of the many operating rooms in this country, the assistant's role has traditionally been filled by a variety of individuals with quite diverse backgrounds as indicated by the following:

1 A qualified surgeon as identified above

2 An MD in a recognized surgical training program

3 An MD without complete surgical training

4 Certified physician's or surgeon's assistants who are not authorized to operate independently

5 A registered nurse or [operating room] technician trained as "scrub nurse" without formal assistant surgical training other than "on the job" or "at the table" experience.

The American College of Surgeons supports the concept that, ideally, the first assistant at the operating table should be a qualified surgeon or a resident in an approved surgical training program.

Attainment of the ideal is recognized as impracticable, and certain individuals without complete surgical training are currently necessary to serve as assistants to qualified surgeons. Certified physician's or surgeon's assistants must make application to the hospital outlining their qualifications and stipulating their requests to assist at the operating table. They shall be responsible to the surgical staff and their performance shall be subject to periodic review.

[The statement by the American College of Surgeons concludes with a discussion of surgery by persons not holding medical degrees, specifically, dentists and podiatrists.]

FINANCIAL ASPECTS

Because the organizational structure of hospitals is still evolving, all who are involved in hospital operations work in a dynamic atmosphere of give and take, and of growth. What is needed today is leadership which can direct the purposes and functions of hospitals toward higher levels of achievement in response to the expectations and needs of society, including fiscal responsibilities. The current hearings in Congress on cost containment in health services are focusing attention on this aspect.

The problems are basically those of adjusting means to ends. These examples illustrate the impact of this type of problem: the myriad of paperwork that results from the various federal programs; third-party payers' requirements for documentation increase the paperwork, and add to the numbers of employees and types of equipment needed to do the work. Educational programs in hospitals are under scrutiny to determine their net costs, balancing actual dollar outlays against the intangible benefits and contribution to services that students make in the process of learning. Having determined costs, they must then establish priorities on which programs to maintain, and how best to fund them. The technology of medicine has grown in the sophistication and consequent expenses of obtaining and maintaining equipment. The temptation to invest in more equipment to offer more services than one's neighbor institution—keeping up with the Joneses—is potent, and calls for hard decisions to be made.

In many respects, hospital administrators are not prepared to deal with these problems, and the frequently cited inability of hospital organizations to operate on a cost-effective basis as do other business organizations adds to the problem. One response to the demand for sound fiscal management has been to contract for hospital management with firms such as American Medicorp, Hyatt Medical Services, American Medical International, or Hospital Affiliates. Writing in *Medical Dimensions,* Gantz[9] notes that "management companies offer more than financial expertise—the area in which most hospitals tend to be weak. They'll also provide total management direction. They can overhaul a hospital's personnel structure, for example, making sure key staff members have the clear lines of communication that will allow them to function properly. And they'll review each individual department to see that the quality of care it delivers meets standards of both the community and the corporate home office."

The criticism that management contracts are strictly commercial in the sense of being interested only in making a profit, is answered by a philosophic principle and a contract provision. The principle is that "there is something that transcends economy, and that is the practice of medicine." In the contract, there is a stipulation that the board of trustees has veto power and thus has a right to intercede when necessary.

Hospital organizations may be influenced by organized interest groups and by government agencies. The chief internal influence among the interest groups is that of health professional societies. Most major, and some minor, health services have their professional organization at national, state, and local levels. The aspirations of these societies for their members will have profound effects on hospital function and organization.

Externally, labor unions, community health groups, and the "third-party" agents of payment for hospital services are important influences. Labor unions have already made some headway in organizing hospital employee groups. Community health groups can influence decisions regarding services to be offered and how they can best be coordinated with community-wide programs. Insurance carriers can and do influence the quality and range of care provided—both of prime importance to hospital administrators.

Governmental influence is ubiquitous not only in the range but in the types of programs. Medicare is the most obvious, making access to health care possible for more people. The affirmative action requirements influence employment practices. Support for educational and research programs, by grants to institutions and individuals, can determine which area has priority in the development of new programs and the expansion of established programs. The Health Services Agencies have the impact on individual institution facilities and programs. The Secretary of DHEW in late 1977 testified that the number of federal programs involving regulatory agencies was at least 380, and perhaps as many as 1,000. With the bureaucratic penchant for paperwork, there is little trouble in assuming that, with such numbers of programs, records, documents, and correspondence have proliferated. In fact, this has become such a nettlesome problem that a special President's Committee on Reduction of Paperwork was appointed to address the issues involved and make recommendations for improvements. The degree of success in implementing its recommendations is yet unknown. Many have little hope for improvement.

Metcalf notes that "malpractice has become one of the most significant constraints affecting the health care system," identifying four factors in the upsurge of costs even though "negligence has probably not increased." He discusses the four factors as leads to finding solutions through organizational development approaches. The factors are: "the consumer revolution; the legal rights explosion; high-expectation technology; and the system's impersonal complexity, which can cause patient disappointment in a faceless technological system." He urges recognizing consumerism as an ally, a basis for the hospital's existence rather than a hindrance. In answer to his question "What action will reduce risk?" Metcalf proposes the following:

Assessment of risk factors to determine the frequency and patterns of incidents, and proactive correction.

Orientation to standards, so that all employees know what is expected of them. Metcalf recommends positively stated standards. Negative standards (thou shalt not) "require surveillance and protective behaviors. . . . Positive standards reflect concern for professional behaviors in process-oriented care."

Skills training to expose shortcuts and bad habits, which are the leading causes of incidents of poor care.

Continuing education that includes not only individual professional growth, but organizational development.

SUMMARY

The organizational structure and functions of hospitals are a complex of internal and external interacting forces that go beyond the dimensions of the usual organization in that the fundamental goal is quality care for the individual, oftentimes with the added burden of "whatever the cost." By their very nature, the problems attendant to achieving this goal are continuous and require maximum understanding on the part of everyone involved if balance is to be maintained.

REFERENCES

1 American Medical Association, "General Principles of Medical Staff Organization," Chicago, December 1964.

2 American Medical Association, "Report on Physician-Hospital Relations," Chicago, June 1964.

3 Bethel, Tom, The Need to Act. *Harper's,* November 1977, pp. 34–40.

4 Brown, Esther Lucile, "Newer Dimensions of Patient Care: Improving Staff Motivation and Competence in the General Hospital," Russell Sage Foundation, New York, 1962.

5 Buckingham, W. B., COLD War: Rationale for Criteria to Assess Respiratory Therapy for Patients with Chronic Obstructive Lung Disease, *Quality Review Bulletin,* September 1977, pp. 22–24.

6 Caseley, D. J., Hospital-Physician Relationships and the Public Interest, *Hospitals,* **26:**66–72, June 16, 1962.

7 Darley, Ward, and Anne R. Somers, Medicine, Money and Manpower III: Increasing Personnel, *New Eng. J. Med.,* **276:**1415–1422, 1967.

8 Friedman, J. W., "Doctors in Hospitals, Medical Staff Organization and Hospital Performance," The Johns Hopkins Press, Baltimore, 1971.

9 Gantz, Paula, Fiscal Therapy for Ailing Hospitals, *Medical Dimensions,* October 1977, pp. 19–23.

10 Heydebrand, W. V., "Hospital Bureaucracy," Dunellen Publishing Co., Inc., New York, 1973.

11 "Higher Education and the Nation's Health: Report of the Carnegie Commission," McGraw-Hill Book Company, New York, 1971.

12 Perrow, Charles, The Analysis of Goals in Complex Organizations, *Am. Soc. Rev.* **26:**854–866, December 1961.

13 Rakich, J. S., "Hospital Organization and Management," Catholic Hospital Association, St. Louis, 1972.

14 Smith, Harvey L., Two Lines of Authority: The Hospital's Dilemma, in E. G. Jaco (ed.) "Patients, Physicians and Illness," The Free Press of Glencoe, New York, 1958, pp. 468–477.

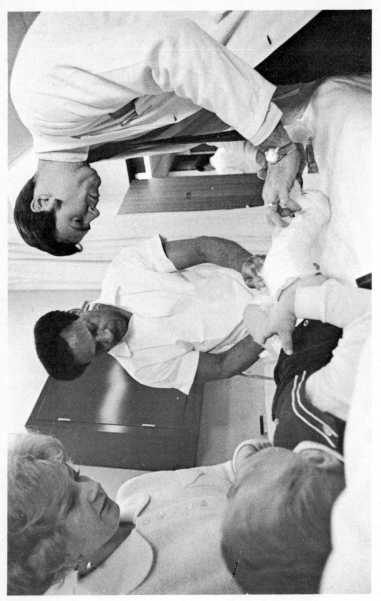

Four members of the health team. (*Courtesy of Bill Rogers.*)

7

HEALTH SERVICES
PERSONNEL

One result of the knowledge explosion has been a necessary increase in medical personnel who can be grouped by the specialized knowledge and skills important to health care activities. The techniques and instruments developed in response to the new knowledge are extremely important, for they have affected the staffing patterns and content of educational programs of many of the health services and precipitated the development of new health occupations. The practice of both medicine and dentistry has developed into subspecialties, and both are becoming more dependent on the services of additional personnel in the diagnosis and treatment of disease. Professional status is yet to be accorded some of these specialized services—a sore point with those denied it. Referring to these essential professions as "ancillary medical services," "paramedical professions," and "health-related services" only reinforces their ambiguous and unstable position in the world of medicine. The term "allied health professions" has become the most common one, largely because of its use in federal documents and acceptability among federal groups.

There is still a long way to go before we reach the greater medical profession Fox[4] looks forward to. Much of the problem lies in the tendency to confuse prestige with exclusiveness—and to bar all others. Also perpetuating the status quo is the traditional legal obligation and right to practice medicine or dentistry.

PROFESSIONS AND PROFESSIONALISM
Definitions

Many definitions of profession have been written through the years, one of the best being that of Supreme Court Justice Brandeis. "A profession is an occupation for which preliminary training is intellectual in character involving knowledge and learning as distinguished from mere skill; which is pursued largely for others and not merely for one's self; and in which financial return is not an accepted measure of success."* Since human need never accommodates itself to the complete convenience of schedules, the professional spirit of service will require a willingness to sacrifice time.

Greenfield's[5] comments on the role of professionalism are of interest as points of view and as definitions.

> The importance of professions in health services cannot be underestimated. No other industry contains such a large number of different types of professions at such different levels of skills. Whether the majority of occupations constitute "true" professions in the sociological sense is unimportant here; the importance lies in the use of the professional model by the members of the occupation and in the effect on the industry of the use of this model.
>
> The justification for professionalism is that the worker has unique competence to deal with a given process, structure, or situation which is important to the community but potentially dangerous in the hands of an incompetent. Because of the supposed unique competence involved, control over the profession should be in the

---

*Remuneration must be ample enough for living expenses and continued professional growth and contributions. It would be unrealistic, and unjust, not to have this essential excellence confirmed and safeguarded by proportional monetary rewards.

hands of the professionals. The three most important aspects of control are *training* new members; *certifying* the competence of those allowed to practice; and *regulating* the quality of practice of the members.

In 1962, the Eastman Kodak Company's advertisement in leading professional magazines was addressed to the concept of professionalism. It contains the essence of the goals of a professional person, and the means to achieve them:

> Professionalism and chance have little in common.
>
> Professionalism is created—built on purpose and devotion.
>
> Professionalism is experience, the total of it. Like a bank account, it grows upon "deposits." Year-upon-year deposits with all the sacrifice of investment of self.
>
> Professionalism is competence to perform, regardless of convenience, fatigue—or luck.
>
> For the true professional, the better he becomes, the higher the standard.
>
> Each patient depends upon medical professionalism. Skill long practiced, experience long ready. Standards long honored.

The American Personnel and Guidance Association, through its Ethics Committee,* compiled a code of Ethics which includes a description of the marks of a profession. The code was published in the October 1961, issue of *Personnel and Guidance Journal.* It is an excellent statement of what separates a profession from an occupation or vocation:

> **1** Possession of a body of specialized knowledge, skills, and attitudes known and practiced by its members.
>
> **2** This body of specialized knowledge, skills, and attitudes is derived through scientific inquiry and scholarly learning.
>
> **3** This body of specialized knowledge, skills, and attitudes is acquired through preparation, preferably at the graduate level, in a college or university as well as through continuous in-service training and personal growth after completion of formal education.

*Members were Seth Arsenian, Chairman, Lee D. Brown, Robert Callis, Warren Findley, Correne E. Gateley, and Thomas Magoon.

4   This body of specialized knowledge, skills, and scholarly inquiry is constantly tested and extended through research.

5   A profession has a literature of its own, even though it may, and indeed must, draw portions of its content from other areas of knowledge.

6   A profession exalts service to the individual and society above personal gain. It possesses a philosophy and a code of ethics.

7   A profession through the voluntary association of its members constantly examines and improves the quality of its professional preparation and services to the individual and society.

8   Membership in the professional organization and the practice of the profession must be limited to persons meeting stated standards of preparation and competencies.

9   The profession affords a life career and permanent membership as long as services meet professional standards.

10   The public recognizes, has confidence in, and is willing to compensate, the members of the profession for their services.

Roles of professionals are a basic consideration and, as Lysaught[8] points out, it is important that roles that interact (as many do in the health professions) be defined in context, rather than unilaterally. He refers to congruence in role definition; for example, there is no teacher role without a learner role. In health professions, for example, the radiologist and the radiologic technologist roles are interacting and interdependent (i.e., congruent), and for either group to define roles independently is unrealistic, and carries the risk of being unacceptable to either or both professions.

Schein[10] raises another important point in discussing the role of the professional, which is in the process of changing because of changes in society. "Since the essence of professionalism is the delivery of service in response to client need, it becomes critical if the professional is to retain his sense of professional identity to identify clearly on whose behalf services are being rendered." There are, according to Schein, three possible clients: immediate, intermediate, and ultimate. The immediate client can be the hospital or other institution that pays the salary of the professional. The intermediate client is the physician who requests the service for his or her patient. The ultimate client is, of course, the patient. Schein points up the issues involved in such definitions of the client by posing questions which may be useful as guides for developing solutions.

> Which one or more of the clients does the professional define as his real client? If the needs of immediate, intermediate, and ultimate clients are in conflict with each other, how does the professional reconcile these conflicts? If the ultimate client is not the one who pays the professional fees, can his interests be properly represented? If professional standards or ethics are to be applied to client-professional relationships, how are these to be applied if they differ for different client systems? Can a professional work for a multiple-client system?

NEEDS AND EXPECTATIONS OF HEALTH PROFESSIONALS

Being human, the members of the health professions have the basic psychosocial needs common to all people: social approval (status), sense of accomplishment, sense of importance of the job, security—all contributing to self-actualization. Self-actualization, the development of a close fit between the concepts of the real self and the ideal self, is best brought about when there are opportunities to exercise intelligence and skills in a meaningful context that gives a sense of completeness. Obviously, with different persons in different situations, there are as many variations as there are differences in personality.

For health professionals, satisfying the needs of self-actualization is accomplished in service that is concerned with just such needs in those whom they serve. The intertwining of these common threads can have orderly, productive results, but sometimes can lead to tangles that frustrate efforts to deliver care effectively. The unique and, at times, burdensome task of all health professionals is to reduce tangles to a minimum. Herein lies one of the satisfactions to be derived from service in health care.

Social Approval

Social approval or its synonym, status, is accorded by both the public (society) and fellow workers among all groups in the health field. When it is withheld by coworkers from those whose self-concept puts high value upon it, there is a considerable expenditure of energy in attempting to win status, or worse, there is "war." As Merton[9] points out,

> Every profession is to some degree surrounded by a zone of
> ambiguity—The trouble with this zone of ambiguity is not that it is a
> no man's land, but that it seems to be everyman's land. And some-
> times this leads to undeclared war between adjacent occupations.

Apart from the almost automatic status the physician enjoys, there
is not yet any sure status for other health professionals. The patterns of organization and responsibility have not evolved into a
well-defined structure. It is in the working out of these patterns that
health care is affected, particularly on the individual, person-to-
person, basis. The "war" catches the patient as an innocent by-
stander, at its worst making that individual the bone of contention
instead of the focus of coordinated effort for her or his betterment.

Sense of Accomplishment
Work is socially approved and rewarding when well done. When
the sense of accomplishment is lacking, it is common to find the
individual or group frustrated and easily fatigued. Important elements of the combination of factors leading to a sense of accomplishment are having sufficient autonomy to make decisions, and
authority commensurate with responsibilities. In too many instances, autonomy and authority are not granted to the degree appropriate to the functions of the newer members of the "greater
medical profession," and as a result levels of productivity are minimal, to the detriment of comprehensive health care. This situation
should change as the team concept gains ascendancy. This should
bring about satisfactions of the need for a sense of importance of
the job as well.

THE HEALTH PERSONNEL PICTURE

The common means of quantification in any enterprise are expenditures and numbers of personnel involved. The health delivery
system is classified as an industry and, as such, is the third largest
in the national economy, and growing rapidly. A comparison of
total public and private expenditures for health care reveals the
magnitude of this industry, and its growth.

   This growth is not primarily related to population growth nor
to shifts in needs (although these are, of course, factors). Rather, it
reflects the phenomenon of the stratification and centrifugation of

Table 7-1 Estimated Number of Persons Employed in Selected Occupations within Each Health Field: 1974

Health field	Number	Health field	Number
Administration of health services	48,200	Nursing and related services	2,319,000
Anthropology and sociology	1,700	Occupational therapy	14,000
Automatic data processing	4,500	Opticianry	12,000
Basic sciences*	60,000	Optometry	25,200
Biomedical engineering	12,000	Orthotic/prosthetic tech.	3,300
Chiropractic	16,600	Pharmacy	132,900
Clinical laboratory services	172,500	Physical therapy	26,100
Dentistry & allied services	279,800	Podiatric medicine	7,100
Dietetic/nutritional services	72,700	Psychology	35,000
Economic research	400	Radiologic technology	100,000
Environmental sanitation	20,000	Respiratory therapy	18,500
Food and drug services	47,900	Secretarial/office services	287,000
Health and vital statistics	1,350	Social work	38,600
Health education	22,750	Special rehabilitation services	12,250
Health information & communication	8,950	Speech pathology/audiology	27,000
Library services	10,300	Veterinary medicine	33,500
Medical records	60,000	Vocational rehabilitation	17,700
Medicine and osteopathy	362,700	Miscellaneous health services	323,950
Total		4,690,250	

*Does not include physical scientists.

Source: U.S. Department of Health, Education and Welfare: *Health Resources Statistics, 1975*. U.S. Government Printing Office, 1976:9-12.

Table 7-2 Personal Consumption Expenditures for Medical Care, Hospital Services and Physician Services (in billions of dollars)

Year	Total medical care		Hospital services		Physician services	
	Expenditures	Cumulative % increase	Expenditures	Cumulative % increase	Expenditures	Cumulative % increase
1960	$ 22.7	—	$ 8.5	—	$ 5.6	—
1965	33.5	48%	13.2	55%	8.4	50%
1970	60.2	165	25.9	205	13.4	139
1974	91.3	302	41.0	382	19.7	252
1975	105.7	366	48.2	467	22.9	309
1976	120.4	430	55.4	552	26.3	370

Note: Figures exclude expenditures in all governmental owned hospitals and nursing homes.
Source: *Social Security Bulletin.* **40:**3–22, April 1977.

functions among the health services, and the burgeoning of scientific and technological developments. Stratification has occurred as both the volume and variety of specific services have increased, leading to the establishment of hierarchies of professional, technical, and supportive personnel. Centrifugation has occurred as it has been determined that functions that were part of those of a particular professional group could be adequately (and sometimes better) performed by less highly educated or trained personnel. The result of this stratification and centrifugation has been the increasingly deplored fragmentation of health services and personnel. What appears to be a rather extreme example is seen in the recent announcement of an associate degree program for the "Extracorporeal Technician," which is described functionally as "operation of heart-lung bypass equipment." This is also an example of another often-deplored, dead-end, confined occupation, i.e., one where there is neither upward nor lateral career mobility potential. This is because it is machine-dependent, and like all machines, is vulnerable to obsolescence in a relatively short time, and even to displacement by newer approaches or techniques for dealing with the problems it now solves.

A listing of health occupations by primary title adds up to 180 types; by secondary titles, the total is 500. Secondary titles may be alternatives, or specialties. In the latter, for example, 57 specialties in medicine and 26 in nursing are listed. Given these data, it is small wonder that territorial "rights" and struggles for status, licensure, and accreditation/certification assume so much importance in the health care area.

Another major problem is providing accurate, solidly based data on personnel needs and employment opportunities. A combination of methods for estimating requirements has been used including surveys concerning budgeted vacancies, ratios to total population, perceived needs, ratios of patient populations, requirements per unit of service, and staffing patterns. Increases in the supply of workers are determined by both predictable and non-predictable factors, among them output of formal training programs, labor market conditions, attrition rates among employed workers, substitutability between health occupations, substitution of nonhealth workers for health workers, and career choices.

Table 7-3   Persons Employed in Selected Health Occupations in the United States, April 1970 (percents in parentheses)

		Racial/ethnic category	
Occupation	Total[1]	Total minority[1]	Black
	Number of persons employed		
Physicians (M.D. & D.O.)	279,658	19,411 (6.9)	6,002 (2.1)
Dentists	92,563	3,739 (4.0)	2,363 (2.6)
Optometrists	17,490	294 (1.7)	148 (0.8)
Pharmacists	110,331	4,757 (4.3)	2,782 (2.5)
Podiatrists	5,956	255 (4.3)	215 (3.6)
Veterinarians	19,041	167 (0.9)	104 (0.5)
Registered nurses	835,797	79,829 (9.6)	65,224 (7.8)
Dieticians	40,225	8,729 (21.7)	7,366 (18.3)
Health administrators	84,416	4,731 (5.6)	3,918 (4.6)
Clinical laboratory tech- nologists, technicians	118,264	15,145 (12.8)	11,021 (9.3)
Dental hygienists	17,458	519 (3.0)	301 (1.7)
Health record administra- tors, technicians	10,946	724 (6.6)	547 (5.0)
Radiologic technologists, technicians	52,566	4,078 (7.8)	3,542 (6.7)
Dental laboratory technicians	26,810	2,311 (8.6)	1,455 (5.4)
Opticians, lens grinders/ polishers	27,844	1,434 (5.2)	1,192 (4.3)
Dental assistants	90,497	4,415 (4.9)	4,415 (3.5)
Lay midwives	914	375 (39.9)	375 (39.9)
Practical nurses	235,546	53,836 (22.9)	51,094 (21.7)
Nursing aides, orderlies, attendants	723,567	192,199 (26.6)	183,398 (25.3)

[1]Includes other races not shown separately.

Source: Health of the Disadvantaged: Chart Book, U.S. Department of Health, Education, and Welfare, Public Health Service, Health Resources Administration, Office of Health Resources Opportunity. DHEW Publication no (HRA) 77-628. September 1977, p.95. (Data base, U.S. Census population, 1970; U.S. Bureau of the Census, Occupational Characteristics, PC(2)-7A, 1973.)

Table 7–3 shows the number and percent of persons employed in selected health occupations in the United States by racial/ethnic categories. This table demonstrates one of the problems of assessing the status of personnel, especially at the national level. There is a marked lag between the time when data are assembled and processed, and the time when they are published. This table was pub-

Racial/ethnic category				
American Indian	Japanese	Chinese	Filipino	White
Number of persons employed				
175 (0.1)	1,654 (0.6)	2,608 (0.9)	5,658 (2.0)	260,247 (93.1)
63 (0.1)	674 (0.7)	423 (0.5)	116 (0.1)	88,824 (96.0)
0 —	58 (0.3)	64 (0.4)	24 (0.1)	17,196 (98.3)
127 (0.1)	874 (0.8)	747 (0.7)	140 (0.1)	105,574 (95.7)
0 —	19 (0.3)	21 (0.4)	0 —	5,701 (95.7)
20 (0.1)	0 —	22 (0.1)	0 —	18,874 (99.1)
1,838 (0.2)	2,524 (0.3)	1,242 (0.1)	6,932 (0.8)	755,968 (90.4)
99 (0.2)	364 (0.9)	189 (0.5)	646 (1.6)	31,496 (78.3)
248 (0.3)	349 (0.4)	42 (0.05)	44 (0.1)	79,730 (94.4)
158 (0.1)	642 (0.5)	1,033 (0.9)	1,832 (1.5)	103,119 (87.2)
0 —	88 (0.5)	60 (0.3)	24 (0.1)	16,939 (97.0)
0 —	68 (0.6)	0 —	87 (0.8)	10,222 (93.4)
134 (0.3)	182 (0.3)	58 (0.1)	91 (0.2)	48,488 (92.2)
21 (0.1)	505 (1.9)	128 (0.5)	142 (0.5)	24,499 (91.4)
23 (0.1)	117 (0.4)	23 (0.1)	58 (0.2)	26,410 (94.8)
151 (0.2)	624 (0.7)	227 (0.3)	179 (0.2)	86,082 (95.1)
0 —	0 —	0 —	0 —	566 (60.1)
1,212 (0.5)	479 (0.2)	169 (0.1)	591 (0.3)	181,710 (77.1)
4,125 (0.6)	1,189 (0.2)	374 (0.1)	1,607 (0.2)	531,377 (73.4)

lished in 1977, and is based on the 1970 population census. Even without waiting for publication, there is a significant lag. For example, processing the 1970 census data to obtain occupational characteristics required three years.

EDUCATIONAL PROGRAM ACCREDITATION
General Considerations

The most important organization involved in specialized program accreditation in the health field in terms of numbers and influence is the American Medical Association. Its activities in accreditation are in medicine through the Liaison Committee on Medical Education (with the American Association of Medical Colleges), and in allied health. In contrast to nursing and pharmacy for example, only a few allied health professions maintain independent accreditation functions.

A study[12] of accreditation functions and practices in selected allied health professions, sponsored jointly by the American Medical Association, American Association of Schools of Allied Health Professions and the National Commission on Accrediting, was conducted under the leadership of William Selden. Following publication of the study report in 1972, efforts were made without success to establish a coordinating organization independent of the AMA. A major stumbling block was the problem of funding, although there were also elements of reluctance on the part of the allied health professional organizations involved because of the potential loss of representation, and for some, the unwillingness to abandon the shelter of the AMA.

Two other organizations have significant influence on specialized accreditation, one in the public sector and one in the governmental sector. In the public sector is the Council on Postsecondary Accreditation (COPA) which operates as a peer review organization in maintenance of standards for accrediting agency/body policies, procedures, and personnel. To be recognized by COPA, an accrediting agency must, through documented evidence, substantially meet the provisions that constitute the standards of COPA. Seeking recognition by COPA is voluntary, but since such recognition carries prestige and credibility, many accrediting agencies find it to their advantage to gain COPA recognition.

In the governmental sector, the U.S. Office of Education (USOE), through its Bureau of Postsecondary Education, Division of Eligibility and Agency Evaluation, conducts a program for recognition of accrediting bodies and applying standards (termed criteria) that also address policies, procedures, and personnel. The principal motivating factor of accrediting bodies in seeking USOE recognition is a service to the programs that are accredited, since eligibility for federal funds is determined by the program or institution having been accredited by an organization recognized by USOE.

AMA and Allied Health Program Accreditation

Prior to 1977, the AMA Council on Medical Education was responsible for accreditation of programs in allied health professions, in collaboration with the respective professional organizations concerned, including the medical specialty societies. The AMA House of Delegates acted on the Essentials (standards) for accredited programs. In response to the growing demand for realignment of the power structure, and spurred on by the USOE and COPA requirements for recognition, the AMA House of Delegates took some important steps in December 1976, loosening the grip of organized medicine somewhat, although the AMA power remained at a high level. Approval of Essentials was delegated to the Council on Medical Education, and a new Committee on Allied Health Education and Accreditation (CAHEA) was authorized to replace the Advisory Committee on Allied Health, and to be responsible for accreditation. CAHEA membership was expanded to include two public members, and provision was made for a student member. Currently, CAHEA's membership includes two educators, four allied health professions, five physicians, one administrator, and two public members. The AMA Department of Allied Health Evaluation is the administrative unit to which CAHEA is related.

The work of reviewing program self-evaluation studies and conducting site visits is done by the 23 review committees on behalf of CAHEA, which then acts on the recommendations forwarded by each committee, granting one of the categories of accreditation, or denying accreditation to those programs that do not meet the Essentials. These review committees are constituted in three patterns: (1) all members are from one allied health professional organization, (2) members are from one or two allied health professional organizations and one or more medical specialty groups; and (3) members are from an autonomous agency which is supported by sponsoring and participating organizations. Examples of these three patterns are shown in Table 7-4.

Sponsoring institutions or units offering allied health education programs accredited by the CAHEA include a variety of types,

Table 7-4 Review Committee Structures

Programs	Representation	Professional groups
Occupational therapist Occupational therapist asst.	Occupational therapists	American Occupational Therapy Association
Radiologic technologist	Radiologic technologists Radiologists	American Society of Radiologic Technologists American College of Radiologists
Medical technologist Medical laboratory technician (certificate & associate degree) Histologic technician	National Accrediting Agency for Clinical Laboratory Sciences Medical technologists Pathologists Technologist-administrator Laboratory director 2-yr. Educators 4-yr. Educators Medical laboratory technicians Histotechnologists Microbiologist Public	American Society of Clinical Pathologists American Society for Medical Technology American Society for Microbiology National Society for Histotechnology

as shown in Table 7-5. Table 7-6 lists the titles of programs, number of programs accredited by CAHEA, and the enrollments of students.

The 27 "collaborating organizations" with AMA include 16 medical specialty organizations, of which two include members who are not physicians; 10 allied health professions societies; and the American Hospital Association. The collaborating organizations support their respective review committees and, with one exception, approve Essentials. The one exception is the National Accrediting Agency for Clinical Laboratory Sciences (NAACLS), whose sponsoring organizations (ASCP and ASMT) delegated authority for approval of Essentials to the NAACLS Review Board. Each of the collaborating organizations is represented on the Panel of Consultants, which meets with CAHEA semiannually.

Other specialized accrediting bodies in allied health include the American Bureau of Medical Laboratory Schools (which accredits programs for the medical laboratory technician and medical assistant, primarily in proprietary schools), and societies of various other specialties such as dietetics (American Dietetic Association), medical illustration (American Medical Illustrators), and speech therapy/audiology (American Association of Speech and Audiology).

Table 7-5   Sponsors of Allied Health Education Programs Accredited by CAHEA

Sponsor	Numbers of Programs	Percent of Total
Hospitals & clinics	1,689	62%
Junior/community colleges	467	17
Colleges/universities	307	11
Other	279	10
Medical schools	137	5
U.S. govt. inst.	68	2.5
Special schools	27	1
Proprietary schools	27	1
Blood banks	13	0.5

Source: AMA Allied Health Education Directory, 1976.

Table 7-6 Types of Programs Accredited by CAHEA

Title	Number	Enrollment
Assistant, primary care physician	51	2,025
Cytotechnologist	99	657
EEG technician	2	11
EEG technologist	9	88
Histologic technician	31	80
Laboratory assistant[1]	129	2,374
Medical assistant	123	4,940
Med. asst. pediatrics	2	39
Med. laboratory technician[2]	59	1,495
Med. record administrator	39	1,121
Med. record technician	66	1,681
Medical technologist	678	7,649
Nuclear med. technologist	134	797
Occupational therapist	47	3,880
Operating room technician	50	316
Physical therapist[3]	76	4,910
Radiation therapy tech.	92	322
Radiologic technologist	1,060	16,932
Respiratory therapist	156	4,902
Resp. therapy technician	99	971
Specialist, blood bank	56	126
Surgeon's assistant	2	39
Total	3,068	55,143

[1]To be medical laboratory technician, certificate program in 1978.

[2]Associate degree program.

[3]These figures may change, with the separation of the American Physical Therapy Association (APTA) from collaborating relationships with AMA. APTA is now conducting its own accrediting program.

Source: AMA Allied Health Education Directory, 1976.

CREDENTIALING FOR HEALTH PROFESSIONALS

Credentials for the individual practitioner may be licensure, certification, or registration. Licensure is a statutory credential earned by passing an examination offered by the state. Certification is earned by passing an examination offered by a professional society, for example, the American Occupational Therapy Association or the American Dietetic Association. In these cases, earning certification also qualifies the individual for membership in the society as an additional mark of entry into the profession. Registration may be earned by examination, or may be a matter of maintaining a roster of personnel judged qualified to practice.

With the impetus toward improving health care, recognition that licensure or certification applies at career entry primarily, and may not attest to the individual's continuing and growing competence is common to many professions in addition to those in the health field. Various approaches to ensuring and monitoring continuing competence have been proposed, with mandatory continuing education emerging as the one which appears to serve both ends. In some professional organizations, documentation of prescribed units of continuing education credits has been adopted as a condition of membership. A growing number of state licensing agencies are requiring the same types of evidence for renewal of licenses. Recertification examinations are being considered in some cases, but have not been implemented to date.

CONCLUSION

The issues, problems, and opportunities in health care related to personnel practices, utilization, and education demand careful and

Table 7-7   Health Personnel Licensure

Health care personnel	Number of states requiring license to practice
Administrator, nursing home	49
Clinical laboratory services director	20
Medical technologist	11
Lay midwife	24
Nurse midwife	14
Nurse	50
Optician	19
Physician	50
Physical therapist	50
Physical therapy assistant	16
Practical nurse	50
Psychologist	48
Radiologic technologist	4
Sanitarian	35
Social worker	7
Speech therapist/audiologist	18

Note: The list does not include those in which licensure is required by only one state.

Source: U.S. Department of Health, Education, and Welfare, *Health Resources Statistics, 1975.* U.S. Government Printing Office, 1976.

coordinated strategies for action if high quality of care is to be achieved while at the same time costs are kept at reasonable levels and services are made available to all the public. The guiding principle must be that "the patient is the central imperative."

REFERENCES

1 Allen, Anne S., "Introduction to the Health Professions," The C. V. Mosby Company, St. Louis, 1976.
2 Bronzino, J. D., "Technology for Patient Care," The C. V. Mosby Company, St. Louis, 1977.
3 Code of Ethics, American Personnel and Guidance Association, *Personnel and Guidance Journal,* October 1961.
4 Fox, T. F., The Greater Medical Profession, *Lancet,* **271:**779, 1956.
5 Greenfield, Harry, "Allied Health Manpower: Trends and Prospects," Columbia University Press, New York, 1969, p. 148.
6 Hamburg, Joseph (ed.), "Review of Allied Health Education 1," University Press of Kentucky, Lexington, 1974.
7 Kay, Eleanor, "Health Care Careers," Franklin Watts Inc., New York, 1973.
8 Lysaught, Jerome (ed.), "An Abstract for Action," McGraw-Hill Book Company, New York, 1970, p. 88.
9 Merton, R. K., Issues in Growth of a Profession, in *Proceedings of the 41st Annual Convention of the American Nursing Association,* Atlantic City, N.J., June 10, 1958.
10 Schein, Edgar H., "Professional Education: Some New Directions," McGraw-Hill Book Company, New York, 1972, p. 24.
11 "Socioeconomic Issues of Health, 1977," American Medical Association, Center for Health Services Research and Development, Chicago, 1977.
12 "Study of Accreditation of Selected Health Educational Programs," National Commission on Accrediting, Washington, D.C., 1972.
13 WHO, "Continuing Education of Health Personnel: Report on a Working Group," Copenhagen, 1977.

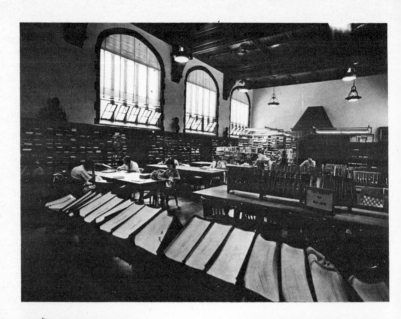

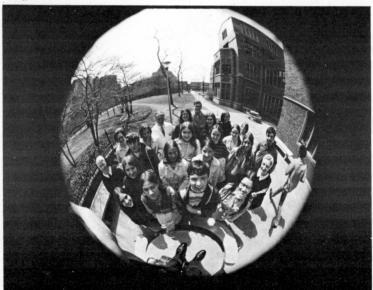

Philosophy is found in books, and finds its meaning in people. *(Courtesy of Bill Rogers.)*

8

TOWARD A PROFESSIONAL PHILOSOPHY

Every science begins as philosophy and ends as art; it arises in hypothesis and flows into achievement . . . the philosopher is not content to describe the fact: he wishes to ascertain its relation to experience in general, and thereby get at its meaning and its worth . . . To observe processes and to construct means is science; to criticize and coordinate ends is philosophy.

Will Durant[3]

PERSPECTIVES IN PHILOSOPHY
Definition

The word philosophy, taken literally, means a love of wisdom. To completely understand that definition, consider the functions of knowledge and wisdom: knowledge is the comprehension of facts; wisdom the evaluation and integration of these facts. Both knowledge and wisdom are essential to the medical scientist, whatever his or her field of activity. There are three operational definitions of philosophy:

1 A study of processes governing thought and conduct; theory or investigation of the principles or laws that regulate the universe and underlie all knowledge and reality.

2 The general principles or laws of a field of knowledge. (This is the basis of the doctor of philosophy degree.)

3 A particular system of principles for the conduct of life; a study of human morals, character, and behavior. (From this definition of philosophy comes our use of the adjective "philosophical," in describing a person who has balance in his reactions, is not easily upset, and takes things in stride.)

IMPORTANCE OF PHILOSOPHY

The third operational definition of philosophy is of great importance in any medical work; it is the framework of the whole of medical services. Durant's comments on the role of philosophy are also pertinent in the context of medical science, for scientists are often accused of concentrating on means to the exclusion of ends, truncating the service to which they subscribe.

A personal philosophy—a philosophy of life—is important because it affects how one behaves. Not many people actually formulate a philosophy in so many words, but each person's actions clearly delineate the characteristics of that person's own particular philosophy of life, and in a real sense are a reflection of the values that an individual holds. The discussion of values clarification given in Chapter 12 offers some guidelines for the process of identifying values and the criteria that may be used in that process.

A PERSONAL PHILOSOPHY

A philosophy of life is basically a framework of values, a hierarchy of importances ranging in a continuum from negative to neutral to positive. Examples of the positive values include justice, charity, prudence, humility, and honesty. But in certain circumstances one's perception influences the weighting of values. What do Americans value in their national life? Is the "democratic way of life" a product, or a process? Many people would define it in terms of the product, individuality: the worth of the individual; opportunity for an individual to fulfill his capacities; individuality rather than autocratic authoritarianism. As a process, the democratic way of life confers on everyone the right to make decisions. Decisions are reflected in activities such as voting (and abstention from voting is a decision in itself, as are all instances of doing nothing); participating in voluntary organizations; writing letters of protest—or praise—to an editor, a senator, or another person whose influence is valued. The democratic process involves the responsibility for its preservation—the responsibility to participate in decision making.

A person's philosophy and character mirror each other, and character, in turn, has much to do with personality, for personality expresses character. Character traits can be positive or negative. Positive traits include loyalty, resourcefulness, tolerance, and courtesy. Most of the character traits adjudged negative by usual standards stem from a lack of concern for others—for example, carelessness, rudeness, selfishness, and jealousy. Even from this short list, the interdependence of character and philosophy is evident: character is the expression, and philosophy the value system determining what is to be expressed.

Philosophy and character, obviously, have much to do with relating to others, and are extremely important in accomplishing personal goals.

For those who work in the world of health care, the values common to daily life take on special significance. The professional person is intelligent, well-informed, and competent; he or she is able to communicate skillfully. In the medical field particularly—though by no means limited to it—professional people are compassionate and tolerant, show courtesy and respect. And, being emotionally mature, they know their own worth and appreciate that of others. They can receive advice, share praise, and give compliments generously. They can also accept criticism or blame when it is due them.

CONCLUSION

Personal philosophy and professional goals provide the criteria for participating in the health care field. What is required is that we fit our knowledge, skills, attitudes, and capacities into the scheme of providing the finest possible comprehensive health care. Implicit in all the medical sciences is the professional workers' belief that beneficial changes in and for society can be accomplished—with their help. In essence, their attitude is expressed in the prayer, "God give me the serenity to accept those things which I cannot change; the courage to change those things which I can; and then, O God, grant unto me the wisdom to know the difference."

The qualifications of the professional person in the health care field are well summarized by Martin.[4]

   1 Vision. With creative talent, he visualizes important attainable goals for himself, and those he serves. This gives him a basis for planning a productive future.

   2 Perspective. With breadth and depth of understanding, he relates himself to his environment and realizes fully how he fits into the total scheme of life. This gives him points of reference and a sense of direction.

   3 Motivation. With inspirational ability, he actuates himself and others to take the necessary logical steps toward the achievement of the established goals. This gives him the initiative needed to undertake the tasks that lie ahead.

   4 Dedication. With thoughtful planning, he wholeheartedly devotes himself to his professional duties and responsibilities. This gives him the persistence needed to complete each task he tackles.

   5 Stability. With calm and patient effort, he persistently, conscientiously, at times, courageously, applies his talents as fully as possible. He takes care not to dilute his efforts by succumbing to hatred, cynicism, fear, or other negative emotions, but attempts to promote good human relationships. Emotional stability gives him quiet dignity which commands respect, fosters close rapport, and makes people attentive to what he says and does.

Philosophy of a Health Service Profession

For any of the health service professions a statement of philosophy expresses the beliefs of its members regarding:

   1 Health—what it is, what it is not

   2 The definition of the health service covered by the particular profession

   3 How the members of the profession function in providing health service

   4 The responsibilities the profession assumes in the planning, delivery, and evaluation of its functions in providing health care—based on the realization that interprofessional cooperation is an integral part of all such functions

The statement of philosophy also prescribes that its members continually maintain the knowledge, skills, and abilities required to provide the quality and quantity of health care consistent with standards of excellence. This is in recognition of the fact that health care is characterized by continuing growth, which demands flexibility to meet the goals it ascribes to. Those in the health care professions must accept their social responsibility for making their goals fulfill the basic human needs of both its practitioners and the public. With understanding and acceptance of their commitment, health professionals can share in creating the growth of humaneness and excellence in the practice of their profession.

For an institution or group, the statement of philosophy describes what the mission is, and how the organizational unit operates to achieve that mission. These, then, lead to the development of specific objectives and the selection of resources and means to implement and evaluate accomplishment, forming a dynamic cyclical system of setting priorities through objectives, implementing the means, and assessing both progress and process for modifications that improve effectiveness.

REFERENCES

1 Bentley, J. E., "Philosophy: An Outline-History," revised edition, Littlefield, Adams & Co., Totowa, N.J., 1966 (paperback).
2 Boyer, Merle W., "Highways of Philosophy," Muhlenberg Press, Philadelphia, 1949 (paperback).
3 Durant, Will, "The Story of Philosophy," Washington Square Press, New York. Paperback edition published by arrangement with Simon & Schuster, Inc., New York, 1961.
4 Martin, Eric W., The Art and Joy of Medical Communication, Address given at the 19th Annual Meeting, American Medical Writers Association, Washington, D.C., Oct. 13, 1962.
5 Vaillot, Sister Madeleine Clemence, Existentialism: A Philosophy of Commitment, *Am. J. Nurs.,* **66**:500–503, March 1966.

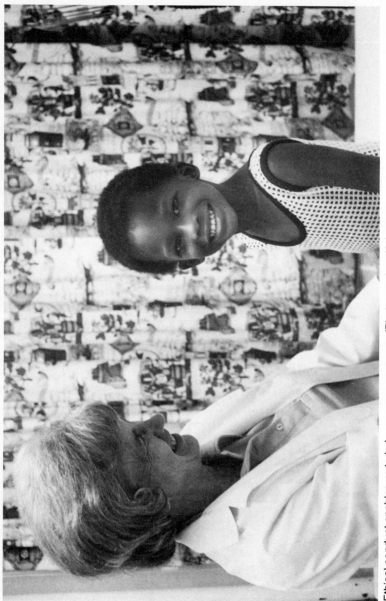

Ethical conduct enables us to help everyone we serve. *(Photo courtesy Univer-*

9

ETHICAL FOUNDATIONS
OF PROFESSIONAL
PRACTICE

Ethics is one of the five fields of philosophical study (logic, esthetics, politics, and metaphysics are the others), but it did not engage the attention of the Greek philosophers of the Ionic period, who were concerned with the problem of substance. Socrates (469–399 B.C.) was the first philosopher to call attention to the importance of inner man as well as nature. "His arguments compelled people to think about questions of right and wrong, justice and injustice, good and evil . . . man could know the nature of the good through reason, but few men were willing to apply rational principles to the study of ethics."[1] Socrates' intense interest in and dedication to the philosophy of ethics made it one of the major fields of inquiry. It is one that has intrigued human beings ever since.

In our context, ethics is the sum of the moral principles and practices necessary to proper care of the sick. However, ethics is part and parcel of everyone's daily life, continually requiring us to make judgments of right and wrong, good and evil, and to decide how to govern our conduct in keeping with those judgments. One's concept of ethics depends a great deal on the beliefs one has about humanity. At one extreme is the belief that we are little more than animals, our conduct governed by deep-seated subconscious drives over which we have no control. Good and evil can have no significance, for we are only biological automatons, not responsible for our actions. Fortunately, this concept is not widely accepted. In medicine, the generally accepted premise is that people have control over their behavior, and it is upon this premise that ethical systems have been developed.

BASIC PRINCIPLES OF MEDICAL ETHICS

Medical ethics is based on a belief in the moral obligations of those who work within the sphere of medicine. Those working in the health care services are under obligation to:

 1 Consistently maintain full professional knowledge and skills
 2 Safeguard the patient against danger to life and health, and avoid unnecessary and unreasonable expense
 3 Observe professional secrecy and honor confidences disclosed in the process of treating the patient
 4 Refrain from engaging in illegal or immoral practices
 5 Safeguard the public and the professions from those who are deficient in moral character and competence

Culpable ignorance and culpable negligence are seen whenever in their lifetimes health professionals fail to maintain standards of learning that enable them to have at their command the knowledge and techniques that improve their contribution to health care—knowledge and techniques that could be life-saving.

Justice, in the context of our list of obligations, means that the health professional will not take unreasonable risks, or risks in which the favorable outcome is highly in doubt. Subjecting the patient to unnecessary or unreasonable expense could be the result of the careless work of a medical technologist and could, for example, necessitate prolonging the patient's hospital stay. The expense can be put not only in monetary terms, but in terms of pain and discomfort.

Sometimes, honoring professional confidences may lead to awkward predicaments. A problem that could be met in ordinary practice occurs when an unauthorized person insists on obtaining information about a patient. This problem arises most commonly when the inquirer is seeking the information by telephone and authority to receive such information cannot be verified. Confidential information may inadvertently be revealed to persons who should not have access to it through careless talk in a public place. A pertinent question is where does professional interest in the scientific elements of the case end and violation of confidence begin?

An example of still another problem involving confidential information occurred when a group of people, in talking about a famous person being treated for urethritis, assumed that the diagnosis was being covered up, and that the patient really had gonorrhea. Drawing the line between violating a confidence and protecting someone's reputation, the one technically informed person in the group pointed out that organisms other than the gonoccocus could cause urethritis.

The definition of what constitutes illegal or immoral practices varies with the cultural or religious context—particularly regarding immoral practices. Certain procedures, such as voluntary sterilization, are immoral in the Catholic context, and this view must be respected. The perennial debates about abortion reflect varying legalities as well as mores.

Even though abortion has been accepted legally, within defined limits, in state laws and by the U.S. Supreme Court, the issue is not resolved in the minds (and hearts) of the many who seek to reverse these decisions. And the issue has spawned still other ethical decisions in the realm of individual rights; for example, whether or not Medicaid benefits may be used to pay for abortions for the poor. The argument against restricting Medicaid benefits is that the poor woman will be denied her right to make an individual choice, whereas the more affluent woman's right will not be abridged. For those who oppose abortion, restricting funds is at least a step in the "right" direction.

Assuming that the public can make judgments about the quality of performance by practitioners in the health care professions is unrealistic, first, because lay people are limited in their knowledge of what to expect, and second, because of the very potent personal element of faith in a given practitioner. In many cases, the practitioner whose performance is judged by peers to be inadequate has been defended to the last ditch by patients or clients whose faith in the person overrides any amount of documented evidence of inadequacy. Nevertheless, health care professionals are obligated to "police" their ranks themselves in order to safeguard the public from those who are incompetent or morally deficient. Here again, the problem is a knotty one, for there must be substantial evidence to support either charge.

The obligation to protect not only the public but one's profession derives from the necessity to maintain the standards of the profession, not letting them be compromised, lest this detract from the whole membership's image and status. A very real challenge is posed for one who knows that a colleague is incompetent. Usually the temptation is to not "blow the whistle," for deciding to do so can be agonizing, and calls for uncommon fortitude. But failure to uphold the law and ethical codes is no less corrupt than their violation. In a healthy society, wrongdoing is protested and the law upheld without fear of involvement or reprisal.

The less obvious, though very real instances of abrogation of responsibilities may be observed in professional practice when the professional person's own attitudes and ability to cope enter the equation. This situation poses a dilemma for the patient's family perhaps more often than for the patient. What of a specialist in oncology, who, when the patient's malignancy has reached the terminal stages, "writes off" the patient almost literally by cutting off conversation or avoiding confrontation of unpleasant developments? An example of this sequence concerns a woman with progressive metastasis of breast cancer. As long as there were specific treatments to be offered, her physician was able to cope. But when the disease went beyond the usual range of treatment and the terminal stage became evident, the physician rather than confronting the patient's needs honestly and forthrightly fell into a pattern of ignoring the patient's questions and search for advice, and frequently referred her to others who were less experienced. The physician's behavior made evident her own inability to face the reality of impending death and her failure to work through the situation *with* the patient.

Ethical considerations arise not only in the clinical setting, but in research as well. For example, Goodfield[11] in writing about her experience in DNA (genetic) research, observes "The problem is that it is so hard to produce rational arguments for one's qualms about DNA research." In the matter of recombinant DNA research, the fact that the scientists themselves voluntarily halted their work and engaged in efforts to evaluate its potential risks to public health is a credit to them in having acted responsibly in the interests of society. From that societally responsible act has come the debate and the guidelines governing recombinant DNA research, though by no means is the controversy completely settled, nor are clear-cut alternatives apparent. As with many ethical issues, there is a cloudy area between the extremes in which the issues must be engaged.

Writing about the other side of the coin of social responsibility, Eisenberg[4] advances the thesis that there are ethical consequences to impeding medical research; that is, supporting excellence in well-chosen research is a social responsibility because of the benefits that are derived from it. Stressing that guaranteeing *absolute* safety is an unobtainable goal and that the public should accept this, he goes on to say:

> I know of no other remedy other than to redouble our effort to explain the nature and justification of well-designed medical research, the calculus of risk and benefit that is an integral part of it, and the design of methods to maximize its potential for gain. If we permit it to be circumscribed with a bureaucracy of regulations so cumbersome as to impede its progress, we incur a risk to society from the restriction of medical science that will far outweigh the aggregate risk to all the subjects in experimental studies.

CODES OF ETHICS

Forerunners of the modern codes of ethics were the oaths ancient physicians took. The oldest one known is the Hindu oath of the physician, which probably dates back to 1500 B.C., and includes many of the points made in today's codes of ethics:

> You must be chaste and abstemious, speak the truth, not eat meat; care for the good of all living beings; devote yourself to the healing of the sick even if your life be lost by your work; do the sick no harm; not, even in thought, seek another's wife or goods; be simply clothed and drink no intoxicant; speak clearly, gently, truly, properly; consider time and place, always seek to grow in knowledge; . . . when the physician enters a house accompanied by a man suitable to introduce him there, he must pay attention to all the rules of behavior in dress, deportment, and attitude. Once with his patient, he must in word and thought attend to nothing but his patient's case and what concerns it. What happens in the house must not be mentioned outside, nor must he speak of possible death to his patient, if such speech is liable to injure him or anyone else. In the face of gods and man, you can take upon yourself these vows; may all the gods aid you if you abide thereby; otherwise may all the gods and the sacra, before which we stand, be against you.

The most familiar of physicians' oaths is attributed to Hippocrates, who lived during the fifth century B.C. Like the Hindu oath, the Greek oath prescribes that

> Into whatsoever houses I enter, I will do so to help the sick, keeping myself free from all intentional wrong-doing and harm. . . . Whatever in the course of practice I see or hear that ought never to be published abroad, I will not divulge, but will consider such things to be holy secrets.

The oath of Aspah and Jochanan is the first known formal pledge of medical ethics among Jews (sixth century A.D.).

In 1948, the World Medical Association adopted an updated wording of the Hippocratic oath:

> At the time of being admitted as a Member of the Medical Profession I solemnly pledge myself to consecrate my life to the service of humanity. I will give to my teachers the respect and gratitude which is their due; I will practice my profession with conscience and dignity; the health of my patient will be my first consideration; I will respect the secrets which are confided in me; I will maintain by all the means in my power, the honor and the noble traditions of the medical profession; my colleagues will be my brothers; I will not permit consider-

ations of religion, nationality, race, party politics or social standing to intervene between my duty and my patient; I will maintain the utmost respect for human life, from the time of conception; even under threat, I will not use my medical knowledge contrary to the laws of humanity. I make these promises solemnly, freely, and upon my honor.

With developments in recent years, there no doubt are those who would be unable to subscribe to this oath because they accept abortion. Note the phrase following the statement on respect for life, "from the time of conception." A modification serving convenience in general use of this oath is simply to delete this phrase.

Haring[12] distinguishes between concepts of professional ethos and codes of ethics. In ethos, attitudes are evident, with tradition as a primary base of customs, experiences, and values, particularly as expressed by those who are respected models in the profession. Codes of ethics, according to Haring, are established standards that relate to the ethos and serve to maintain its values. Smith has identified several criteria by which codes of ethics may be assessed: it states *principles* rather than rules, is specific for the group, includes means to deal with violations (consistent with legal requirements), and is amenable to change when appropriate. Purtillo[19] further notes that a code of ethics should "constitute the heart of ethically sound professional practice," and that it cannot be expected to be a comprehensive set of rules covering all situations.

The AMA was founded in 1847, and adopted a code of ethics published in 1803 by the English physician, Thomas Percival. In the AMA code, eight principles, which have been used by many other health professions as a model are identified.

1   The objective of medical practice is to render service to humanity will full respect for the dignity of man.

2   The physician must improve his knowledge and skills, and communicate them to others.

3   The physician will practice a method of healing founded on a scientific basis.

4   The physician will safeguard the public and himself against those physicians who are deficient in moral character or professional competence.

5   The physician may choose whom he will serve.

6 The physician will not dispose of his services under terms or conditions which tend to interfere with or impair free and complete exercise of his medical judgment and skill.

7 The physician will limit his income to service rendered by him or under his supervision.

8 The physician will seek consultation on request, in doubtful or difficult cases in order to enhance medical service.

The viability of any service which deals, as does medicine, with the intimately personal elements of an individual's life is dependent upon the dedication of its practitioners. This has been recognized through the ages, and continues to be the guiding light of truly professional service.

DECISION MAKING INVOLVING ETHICS

Puzzles always come when there is conflict, when there is engagement between differing values or rights requiring accommodation to the needs of society, the needs of the patient, or the needs of the practitioner. Since there are no sets of rules that cover all situations, the primary concerns have to be (1) sensitivity to the very existence of an ethical situation and (2) development of decision making skills in the ethical context.

In her chapter on components of an act that makes a difference, Purtillo identifies four elements: the agent, the circumstances, the intent, and the consequences, each of which may be judged for ethical characteristics. The first step in decision making is to determine whether or not ethics may be involved, followed by use of the principles of an ethical code in determining specific action to be taken. As much, perhaps, as anything, ethical considerations are matters of good conscience, as individually personal as one's signature. What one ascribes to, is attuned to, and is willing to attest to become the basis for action.

REFERENCES

1 Boyer, Merle W., "Highways of Philosophy," Muhlenberg Press, Philadelphia, 1949.

2 "Casebook on Ethical Standards of Psychologists," American Psychological Association, Inc., Washington, D.C., 1967.

3 Catholic Medical Ethics, *J.A.M.A.*, **180:**834–835, June 9, 1962.

4 Eisenberg, Leon, The Social Imperatives of Medical Research, *Science,* **198:**1105–1110, Dec. 10, 1977.

5 Ethics of a Protestant Physician, *J.A.M.A.*, **181:**253–254, July 21, 1962.

6 Exploring Humanistic Health Science Education, proceedings of a conference for faculty at the University of Illinois at the Medical Center, Chicago. Mar. 16, 1977.

7 Frankena, W., "Ethics," Prentice-Hall, Inc., New York, 1963.

8 Goodfield, June, "Playing God: Genetics Engineering and Manipulation of Life," Random House Inc., New York, 1977, p. 169.

9 Goodfield, June, Humanity in Science: A Perspective and a Plea, *Science,* **198:**580–585, Nov. 11, 1977.

10 Haring, Bernard, "Medical Ethics," Fides Publishers Inc., Notre Dame, Ind., 1973.

11 Inglefinger, F. J., Bedside Ethics—Professional or Universal, *N. Eng. J. Med.,* **289:**914, 1973.

12 Jewish Medical Ethics, *J.A.M.A.*, **180:**402–404, May 5, 1962.

13 Maddock, J. W., Humanizing Health Care Services: The Practice of Medicine as a Moral Enterprise, *J. Nat. Med. Assoc.,* **65:**501–504, 1973.

14 Mead, Margaret, The Cultural Shaping of the Ethical Situation, in K. Vaux (ed.), "Who Shall Live?" Fortress Press, Philadelphia, 1970.

15 Medical Research: Statistics and Ethics. A collection of papers presented at the Birnbaum Memorial Symposium, *Science,* **198:**677–699, Nov. 18, 1977.

16 Mohr, James, "Abortion in America. The Origins and Evolution of National Policy," Oxford University Press, London, 1978.

17 Purtillo, R. B., "Essays for Professional Helpers: Some Psychosocial and Ethical Considerations," Charles B. Slack, Inc., Thorofare, N.J., 1975.

18 Roth, Russell, The Dilemmas of Human Experimentation, *Modern Medicine,* **43:**56–61, February 1975.

19 Smith, R. H., "New Directions for Ethical Codes," *Association and Society Manager,* December/January 1974.

20 Veatch, Robert M., "Case Studies in Medical Ethics," Harvard University Press, Cambridge, Mass., 1977.

21 Veatch, Robert M., Human Experimentation: The Crucial Choices Ahead, *Prism,* **2:**58–61, July 1974.

22 Visscher, M. B., Moral Values vs. Scientific Progress, *Modern Medicine,* **43:**62–64, February 1975.

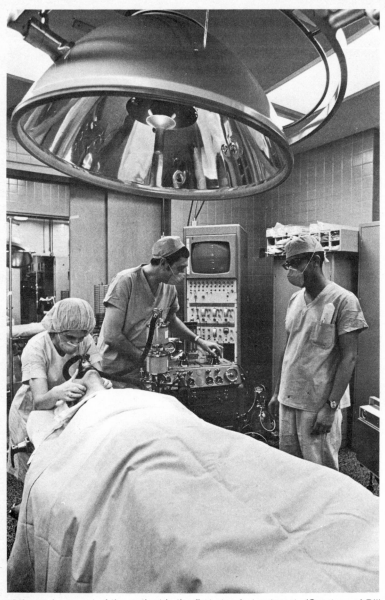
Informed consent of the patient is the first step in treatment. *(Courtesy of Bill Rogers.)*

10

LAW AND PROFESSIONAL PRACTICE

Laws are essential to the harmony of all social groups in order to protect society and regulate those activities that impinge on the rights of individuals and have the potential for harm. Liberty is not license; the first law of conduct must be self-discipline if people are to live fully. The discipline of formal law controls society's behavior and ensures orderly processes of daily living. Law defines the obligations and benefits of prescribed behavior and also the penalties for not conforming to it.

In distinguishing between the imperatives of law and ethics, St. John-Stevas[3] writes:

> Law enforces only those standards of moral behavior indispensable for community existence; morality has no such pragmatic limitation, but calls for conformity with the ideal. The man who limits himself to legal observance may be a tolerable citizen, but has no claim to be

considered a good man of western tradition, much less the good neighbor of Christian thought.

As we shall see, there are other dimensions of law that have important influences on health care and the health care system.

HISTORICAL REVIEW

Although they may not be specifically prescribed and enforced, there are regulations in every social unit accompanied by sanctions against the members of the unit who do not conform. Through mores and taboos, expectations and understanding of what is acceptable conduct, social units maintain discipline. Sanctions applied to those who do not comply include the withholding of approval and, in some cases, ostracism. Primitive peoples in the early history of humanity recognized the need for rules and codes to govern group living, and venerated the "law-givers" and judges who promulgated their laws for them.

The first known formal code of law was formulated by the Babylonian King, Hammurabi, who lived from 2067 to 2025 B.C. Mosaic law is familiar to us from the Hebrew Scriptures. Draco, a Greek of the sixth century B.C., is remembered by the adjective which describes severe and harsh laws—draconian. Emperor Justinian (483–565 A.D.) sponsored the Roman code of law which is the basis for much of European law. Napoleon organized the law of his empire, and his code is common to France, and, in part, to Louisiana and Quebec in modern times.

The American system of laws is based on English common law. Common law is derived from records of cases tried by the King's Court. When Parliament was established in 1295, a legislative body was empowered to write formal laws. These laws, in contrast to common law, are called statutory laws. Our Congress and state legislatures (or assemblies, as they are called in some states) have their roots in the English system, though modified somewhat to fit different needs and a different system, since ours is not a parliamentary system of government.

Interpretation of the law and its enforcement are in the hands of the courts of each political unit making up American government. The jurisdiction of the courts is determined by geography and by the types of cases to be tried.

There are a number of kinds of laws which are categorized as follows:

Civil—negligence, libel and slander, commercial disputes
Contract—agreements between persons and organizations
Common—principles and rules of action
Criminal—offenses (e.g., traffic violations), misdemeanors (e.g., petit larceny, assault and battery), and felonies (major crimes of robbery, murder, and arson)
Martial—law in times of emergency
Military—misconduct in the armed forces
Statutory—the full range of laws enacted by legislative bodies

Statutory laws are those which have the most far-reaching effects. They include authorization of and appropriations for governmental programs such as those promoting health, the Social Security system, taxes, etc. The corollary to statutory laws is the body of regulations that carry out the intent of the legislation. For example, the Illinois General Assembly recently modified the statutory provision for renewal of the physician's license to practice by including a requirement for continuing medical education as a condition of renewal. The regulations developed to carry out the intent of this change specify the details of types of continuing medical education recognized, how the evidence of having participated in such programs is to be presented, the penalties for noncompliance, the appeal mechanism in cases of denial of a renewed license, and the responsibilities of institutions and organizations offering continuing medical education. Regulations must be enacted by the designated agency according to a specific process which includes public opportunities for comment. Once approved, regulations become part of the law and have the force of law. Rules, on the other hand, are not law, but are the means by which administrative agencies carry out their responsibilities in implementing the law.

Another nonlegislative process in which law develops is in judicial opinions relating to specific cases. Judicial opinion has the force of law within the jurisdiction of the particular court in which it originated. The judges interpret general statements in the law, applying legal principles to the specific case. The resulting written opinions are then used to enforce the law within the limits of the particular court's sphere. For example, in interpreting the general statements in the Civil Rights Act, as it pertains to a given case such as racial balance in public schools, the judge hearing the case applies legal principles and develops an opinion that may result in requiring the school board to achieve racial balance by transporting pupils from one school district to another.

As Wing[4] points out, even a cursory acquaintance with legislative action leads to the conclusion that "the law is an important determinant of the public's health and the health care delivery system, and is therefore a means of bringing about change." The health care community of interests is just as concerned with the regulations that are promulgated as it is with the laws passed by legislative bodies such as the United States Congress.

LAW AND HOSPITALS

As indicated in the chapter dealing with the organizational structure of hospitals, the governing board is the legal agent of the hospital. As such, it has powers derived from an act of the state in which it is located incorporating the institution. The incorporation document clearly states the institution's purpose and authority to function. These are: that there will be reasonable care and skill applied in the operation of the institution; that there will be proper use of funds; that the governing board will protect and preserve the property of the institution; that it will provide satisfactory care for patients; that due care and diligence in supervising the activities of the hospital's personnel will be applied; and that a competent medical staff will be maintained. The governing board may delegate these duties in an appropriate manner, with the proper authority to carry out assignments, but it is ultimately responsible before the law for the actions of those delegated.

While the doctrine of immunity for charitable institutions protects charitable hospitals from liability due to negligence of the hospital or its employees, this doctrine is gradually losing court support. It originated from judicial decisions, its first application being in 1876 in Massachusetts, and was followed routinely until the last few years. Two types of liability are applicable to the hospital in cases of negligence: *respondent superior*, and corporate negligence. In *respondent superior* (literally, "let the master respond"), the hospital is liable for negligent acts of its employees. Corporate liability applies to negligence associated with defective equipment, incompetent personnel, or poor maintenance of buildings and grounds. With the shift away from hospital immunity for charitable institutions, the individual becomes increasingly the focus of legal action, as is shown by suits involving malpractice.

Each person who functions in the hospital, particularly professional personnel, must employ every reasonable care in carrying out his or her duties. The definition of "reasonable" is currently determined according to standards common to the given community and will probably be influenced significantly by the work of the Professional Standards Review Organizations (PSRO), since the criteria upon which audits are assessed are quite precise. In cases of malpractice suits where the burden of proof is upon the defendant—all the plaintiff need do is institute the suit. This is based on the principle of law that "the thing speaks for itself." This is in contrast to the requirement in other cases that the prosecution marshal proof of guilt of the defendant. Another aspect in which medical malpractice suits are different is that the statute of limitations, which requires that a suit be brought to court within a certain specified time, is not so limited. Because the hospital is responsible for its employees, it maintains established rules and regulations that the employees must follow explicitly.

Importance of Consent of the Patient

The patient's consent is required before certain treatments or procedures are legally permitted. Performing such procedures without the patient's consent is defined as battery. The proof of consent is a document signed by the patient stipulating that the hospital and its employees may do whatever is necessary in his or her treatment. Only when there is an emergency, a life-threatening situation, can this proof of consent be reasonably ignored. When surgery is involved, hospitals require a second consent document that commonly includes a statement allowing the surgeon to perform procedures that may not have been anticipated but for which the need becomes apparent during the surgical procedure originally consented to. This document is important because the patient, obviously, is not in a condition during surgery to provide the extension of permission. It is a rare patient who does not assume she or he will get competent professional care. The act of coming to the hospital for admission is an implied consent to whatever treatment may be necessary.

Professional persons employed by the hospital must work within the limits of their professional competence. When they are asked to do something that they know, or suspect, is outside the limits of their competence, they should, in order to protect themsevles from culpability if legal action is subsequently taken, state that their competency does not extend to this particular procedure.

One of the most common critical areas of legal responsibility is concerned with identification of the patient and of specimens of any kind removed from him or her for diagnostic purposes. There are two ways in which this is critical: (1) improper identification can result in treatment that is unwarranted, and possibly even life-threatening; and (2) the patient can sue for defamation of character if he or she is mistakenly identified as having a socially condemned disease. A mistake in a laboratory test result, even so simple a one as a misplaced decimal point, can lead to treatment for the wrong condition. Blood for transfusions is extremely vulnerable to misidentification; a transfusion can be life-threatening if the wrong type of blood is administered to a patient.

Recourse to legal means to solve the problem of unwitting transfusion of blood with the potential for infecting the recipient with hepatitis has been taken in the form of requiring the labeling of units of blood drawn from donors who were paid. This has been done in several states, and is based on the findings that "paid donors" are more likely than volunteers to have a higher incidence of hepatitis, and a considerable number of them are not consistently honest in reporting this at the time of the donor screening interview. Although reliable tests are available for many diseases that may be transmitted by the infusion of blood, those for hepatitis have become available only recently.

Consistent with the Fifth Amendment of the Constitution, a test for the blood alcohol level of a person involved in a prosecutable offense such as driving while intoxicated can be interpreted as a form of testifying against oneself, and this must be made clear before the blood sample is obtained. It is a vexing problem, and attempts have been made to solve it through laws specifying that a test for a chemical in the blood is admissible evidence even when obtained without full consent.

Medical Records

For every hospital patient there is a record of his or her hospital course that details the diagnosis, prognosis, treatment, records of tests performed, and progress during the illness for which the patient is hospitalized. These records are legal documents in every sense, and great care is essential in keeping them. Nothing may be erased from the record—when an error in recording is made, the information is struck out and labeled "error." The entire record constitutes confidential information, and the only one who can authorize its release is the patient or, if he or she is a minor or incompetent, someone acting on the patient's behalf. Similarly, photographs may not be taken without written consent. Aside from its legal use, a medical record is useful in research and may be needed in reporting results of research. The requirement before publication is that permission be obtained, and that the case history, etc., be anonymous.

PRECAUTIONS IN CARRYING OUT ORDERS

When an accident happens to a patient as a result of carrying out a physician's order, and should the patient subsequently sue for damages, the court is interested in answers to these questions:

1 Was there a medical order?
2 Was it written or oral?
3 Exactly what was the order given?
4 Was it medically sound, and were the instructions complete?
5 If not, was the error or omission such that a reasonably competent professional person could be expected to question the order before carrying it out?
6 If it was sound and complete, did the person involved carry it out in a reasonably competent manner, i.e., in a manner comparable to the way in which others with adequate training and experience would have handled the order?
7 Was the accident unpredictable and unavoidable?

Depending upon the answers to these questions, the decision of the court will be made. If guilt is determined, the physician alone may be found culpable of malpractice or neglect. Or the person carrying out the order, either alone or jointly with the physician, may be found guilty. The third possibility is that the institution, as a vicarious agent *(respondent superior),* either alone or jointly, is the culprit. If the accident is deemed unpredictable and unavoidable, then no guilt is attached.

In view of this, there are a number of precautions that may be taken by the person who is to carry out the order, so that he or she will have maximum protection against culpability.

1 If the physician gives the order in person:
   a Repeat it back before acting on it.
   b Remind the physician (if needed) to write it on the patient's order sheet before he or she leaves the hospital.
   c Check the order sheet after the physician leaves. If he or she failed to write the order, make a notation in the nurse's notes as to the exact order given, from whom, and what was done about it.

2 If the order is relayed to a second person:
   a If it seems right, carry it out, then make a notation in the nurse's notes as above.
   b If there is a reason to question the order, contact the physician to make sure it was repeated correctly.
   c If the physician is not available in person or by phone, refer to a superior for action.

3 If the order is given on the phone:
   a Write it down, then read it back slowly and clearly, for confirmation.
   b If there is anything about the order that is not fully understood, ask questions until it is understood.
   c Find out when the doctor will be in to write the order; check the order sheet at the proper time, and proceed as in 1c.
   d If an order must be requested from the physician during the night, be sure he or she seems fully awake and understands the situation before proceeding as above.

LICENSURE

The purposes of licensing professional personnel are (1) to discourage the growth of groups that claim the practice specified, but whose members have not had proper education and training; (2) to prevent nonqualified persons from calling themselves professional; (3) to allow reciprocity with those states that already have licensure or registration so that professionals may move and practice without loss of legal status; and (4) to prevent any state from becoming a dumping ground for persons who cannot meet the standards of states requiring licensure or registration.

The benefits to the public accrue from the assurance of receiving competent services; to the medical profession from the availability of quality service in health care; and to the individual patient from the protection against misrepresentation and infringement by nonqualified persons. Licensure laws may define the legal responsibilities of the licensee, define the limits of functions of various categories of workers, and prescribe the educational and practical qualifications of a candidate for licensure. In almost all cases, licensure requires an examination administered by a specified Board; in some cases, the educational programs required are defined, and rules for accreditation of schools are delineated. In all cases, a section of the licensure laws defines the sanctions to be imposed, and the penalties for breaches of the law, as well as for malpractice, are listed.

A license to practice in one of the medical professions is both a legal document and a testament to the privilege society grants the licensee to practice his or her profession. Having been granted the right to practice medicine, the physician is keenly conscious of the responsibilities that this right entails. The final decisions are his or hers in what can, and should, be done for the patient. The physician or dentist enters into a contract with each patient and is committed to act in the patient's interest. If the physician delegates some of his or her responsibility to other professionals, the physician—or the patient—may construe it as a breach of contract. Also, such diffusion of responsibility might be detrimental to the patient.

To some of the health professions personnel, licensure is attractive as a measure of the professionalism for which they strive. In part, this is because the public considers physicians, dentists, and nurses "professionals" by associating licensure with professionalism. A second consideration is that licensure requires professional education and training and thus prevents unqualified persons from being admitted into the professions. This consideration has been abused in some instances where by setting standards that are so restrictive, there is actual control of the numbers of entrants to the pool of professionals, thereby establishing a high–demand, high–salary situation. There is legitimate reason, in such cases, to question the motivation of proponents of such standards, which leads to the conclusion that economics, i.e., controlling the numbers of entrants in order to maintain high levels of earnings and reduce competition for jobs, is the root of their concern.

Legal definitions of responsibilities and limits of practice can establish reasonable grounds for proper development and continuing improvement of standards of a profession, but this argument can be challenged if there is not, in fact, evidence that improvement will result from the licensure law.

REFERENCES

1 Lewis, Ted, Jr., Medicine in Congress: The Incredible Machine and How It Grew, *Prism,* **2:**17–19, January 1974.
2 Saperstan, S. A., Medicine in Congress: How a Bill Becomes Law, *Prism,* **2:**21–23, January 1974.
3 St. John-Stevas, Norman, et al., "Life, Death, and the Law," Eyre and Spotteswoode, London, 1961, pp. 14, 15.
4 Wing, K. R., "The Law and the Public's Health," C. V. Mosby Company, St. Louis, 1976.

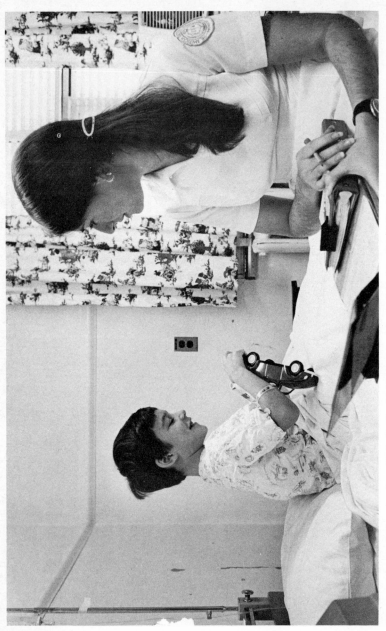

Interpersonal relations begin with individuals. (Photo courtesy of University of Rochester School of Medicine.)

11

INTERPERSONAL RELATIONS

The rapid manner in which the specialties developed within the broad framework of medicine required the interest and energy of a great many people. With maturity, each of the specialties may be expected to, and should, devote more energy to the development of professional cross-fertilization and cooperation. True enough, proper self-regard is necessary—in both individuals and professions—but not to the extent that it causes the dissension and discord that are destructive to teamwork.

The impact of specialization in the health care world has emphasized the differences rather than the similarities of professionals in their interpersonal as well as their work relationships. Particularly in group situations, these individual differences must be used constructively, for each person's unique contribution is necessary to the functioning of the whole. To illustrate in a simple material way, think of the function of the hook and eye. Neither can function properly without the other; it is the combination of the two which fastens securely. So should each specialist's contribution combine with others in a functional way to accomplish the purposes of comprehensive health care. Concepts of team development are discussed in the following chapter. Here, the discussion will focus on some general considerations and principles in interpersonal relations.

A LOOK AT PERSONALITY

Interpersonal relations begin with individuals, then proceed to their integration into groups. The interaction of personalities influences what individuals bring to groups, and what groups give to individuals.

Definitions of Personality

Few other words in our language have such fascination for everyone as does personality. Most popular meanings fit into these classifications: social skill and adroitness; effectiveness in provoking reactions from a variety of persons under different circumstances. The qualities of the first classification are what the so-called charm schools try to teach. The second classification may be translated into a phrase such as "the impression created on others." In this instance, terms such as aggressive, submissive, cheerful, dull, strong, weak, modify the word personality. It is difficult to generalize about personality because its definition depends upon the context or upon the framework of a choice of personality theory. Perhaps the simplest definition of personality is the organization of traits within the individual relative to his environment.

Hypothesizing about the behavior of people conditions an approach to a proposition or problem so that we can succeed in achieving our purposes. Aware of it or not, we are all "practical" psychologists.

Another common tendency is to oversimplify and attach labels to people. The familiar stereotypes are not necessarily valid. Is the woman French? Then she must be romantic. Is the man British? Then he must have a dull sense of humor, be pedantic, and very class-conscious. Members of the health care professions do not escape stereotype labeling; for example, the nurse as a surrogate mother. It is in stereotyping that some of the most important expectations find their bases, bases that are at times established on shifting sands. Stereotyping is largely a reflection of a lack of understanding, and involves generalizations that are often vulnerable to being refuted, rather than confirmed.

ATTITUDES

Actions are governed, to a large extent, by attitudes. An attitude may be defined as an enduring system of positive or negative evaluations, emotional feelings, and tendencies toward action (pro or con). Attitudes about people are based on beliefs about them, feelings toward them, and a disposition to respond to them. By knowing the attitudes of people, it is possible to do something about predicting and controlling their behavior. Politicians use attitudes in predicting how people will vote, and often expend great effort to make the voters' attitudes conform to the goals of the party—or else the party's goals are shifted to conform to the prevailing attitudes of the voters. Attitudes are involved in responses to every phase of living, and, as a rule, are not isolated on a one-to-one basis, but appear in clusters of related elements. Important in the formation of attitudes is how well an attitude serves to fill a need for status, respect, acceptance, or security. Attitudes that help to satisfy these needs are sometimes consciously cultivated.

Attitudes are shaped by the information to which one is exposed, whether it is accurate or spurious. Lacking a so-called authoritative source, most people invent "facts" if the want which is supplied by a particular attitude has functional necessity. Thus, the validity of attitudes depends upon the reliability of sources of information, the range of personal experiences, and the degree to which major wants are adequately satisfied.

In many respects, attitudes reflect personalities. Other things being equal, it is easier to change attitudes if the new attitude is consistent with personality. The naïve person has less stability in his or her attitudes. Attitudes which have strong social support through group affiliations are difficult to change because of group members' tendency to cling to attitudes endorsed by the group, in order to remain in good standing. A change in actions or behavior may come about through coercion by an external force; for example, by contact with the object of the attitude, or by law, or through circumstances. Authority, social mores, or rewards may influence people to play roles that express attitudes that are contradictory to their inner evaluations, but, in the process of role playing, their actual attitudes may change.

GROUPS

Every institution has its individual history, formal regulations, and informal customs, which make it distinctive. Within an institution, such as a hospital, are individual departments containing smaller units. It is in this kind of setting that our interpersonal relations are conducted.

The groups to which one belongs have a great deal of influence on success in reaching goals that have been chosen as worthwhile. The groups may be formal or informal, their influence negative or positive. Each group has norms and goals, and the means of keeping its members within bounds through sanctions, penalties, or ostracism. Group membership serves many needs, especially that for support, and, with support, the participants are better able to accomplish personal goals and contribute to those of the group.

Operationally, a group comprises several persons who are working together, in a person-to-person setting, to achieve goals. In the health care professions, these goals are focused on health care in the context of a special service coordinating with other special services. On this person-to-person basis within a group, the benefits that accrue are related to the enrichment possible from the exchange of knowledge and experience, clarification and constructive modifications of ideas, and interest in others, all of which help in finding solutions to problems. To realize these benefits, it is important that all members of the group be willing to make their own unique contributions.

To make the most of what the members may contribute, a good leader is essential. The emergence of a member as a leader usually comes about naturally, although there are times when he or she may have this role assigned. The qualities of leadership that mark a good leader are the abilities to (1) guide (not push) the group so that it keeps on target, in discussions and actions; (2) help create and maintain a comfortable atmosphere; (3) focus diverging opinions and solutions on the problem at hand so that a consensus can produce the desired result in decisions reached; (4) help carry out the action required by these decisions. The group leader succeeds best when it is clear that he or she believes in the members and respects them as persons. It is important that the leader offer his or her services to the group, not impose them arbitrarily.

Important as the leader is, nothing would be accomplished without good group members. Within groups there are qualities which result in productivity or frustration. These qualities are evidenced by the roles members play in deliberations and action. Productivity will be more likely if there are self-starters who offer ideas and points of view to help generate and maintain purposeful activity. Others may assist the leader in keeping the activities well-focused on the problem at hand. Each member should be a contributor.

The qualities of group members that frustrate action are aggression, obstruction, domination, or lack of concern. Aggressive members tend to use their energies in destructive opposition. The obstructionist is one who cannot be moved to agree despite arguments to the contrary. In dominating, a member tries to impose his or her will to make others do what he or she wants done. Lack of concern is evidenced by carelessness, low-level interest, or a flippant attitude.

In order to accomplish its goals, the group must take several steps, each involving the ultimate decision about a course of action. The first step is one of definition. It involves getting at the source rather than the symptoms of the problem; determining which factor(s) are of greatest importance; setting up realistic objectives; and identifying the limitations within which the solution must operate.

The second step is analytical, in which a number of questions must be answered, the first being who has to do what in order to put the decision into operation. The second has to do with obtaining accurate information, and determining what estimates might be needed in areas where information is not available.

On the basis of the first two steps, a tentative decision may be reached, but it is wise to have alternatives available, and from those offered, to choose the best decision. To translate the decision into action, the final operation is effective communication so that all persons involved understand what the decision is, and the necessary steps that must be taken to carry it out.

Inability of a group to reach a decision may be due to a single factor or a combination of factors. These include (1) fear of the consequences, in which the prevailing attitude is "if we don't go to bat, we won't stand a chance of striking out"; (2) a dilemma imposed by divergent loyalties expressed, for example, "if we go along with this decision, we'll pull the rug out from under Joe, and after all he is important to us in other ways"; (3) differences of opinion that result in a collision course; and (4) poor leadership resulting in an impasse.

To develop effective group work, it is wise to evaluate the action as it is played out during the process of arriving at a solution. It can be helpful, in this regard, to have an observer who can judge the important elements of the process. Review of the proceedings should enable the leader to determine (1) the degree and kinds (ideational, emotional) of interaction; (2) the potential of the interaction to stimulate formation of ideas; (3) areas of conflict and hostility which need defusing; (4) adequacy of communication, and (5) goal-direction.

These principles of group dynamics may be fruitfully applied to groups within a department or to those involving persons from a variety of departments. It is also possible to apply them to one-to-one interpersonal relations, for they are just as meaningful at this level.

COMMUNICATION

By definition, communication is a process of passing information and understanding from one person to another. It always involves at least two people, a sender and a receiver. It also involves two elements, information and understanding. The media for communication are extremely varied. They may be words, pictures, action, or inaction. Supporting elements are, for example, the tone of voice, gestures, purposeful silence, or unexplained action.

Even an accurate report of facts can be altered by the reporter's choice of adjectives, particularly if he uses emotionally loaded words. Such descriptions as "Winston Churchill, wholly

British, half American," or the *Time* magazine report of a luncheon speech in connection with a reference to the possible menu as "a little hunk of baloney" convey more than the mere reporting of events.

Pictures may be used to convey meanings without words. Political comment can be made by the cartoonist who is a master at this, such as in the cartoon depicting the AMA as Scrooge in relation to Medicare. An unflattering photograph of a public figure may be chosen by a newspaper editor to stimulate or reinforce negative views.

Uses of Communication

Primarily, communication is a means of accomplishing objectives, personal and professional. The range of objectives is limitless—from getting to know a loved one to "selling" a political candidate. In education, communication is the teaching/learning tool. Socially, it is a means of identifying with a group, obtaining status, or unity. To the leaders of the nation, it is a means of obtaining support for their policies through explanation and appeals. In business, it is a means of selling goods and services through advertisements that create a sense of need in potential buyers, and offer information about the product's qualities.

Communication as a Function of Professional Competence

In any profession, communication is essential to accomplishment. One person must report to another in order to coordinate functions or to provide information essential to performance of duties. For example, the nurse must provide accurate requisitions to other departments if they are to complete the orders. Conveying specific knowledge to others is an important function of communication and can improve understanding of problems each person or department faces.

Professional competence is enhanced by information provided by the written word in journals, the spoken word at professional meetings, and in private conversations during which knowledge and experience are shared.

Barriers to Communication

Status and position can bar communication if the one to whom it is addressed rebels against authority. Social levels are important: the poor man may reject the rich man's message by tuning him out.

Language may be a barrier if the sender and receiver have different concepts of the meaning of the words used. It has been said that words don't mean, people mean.

If there is a built-in resistance to change, there will be no communication, since the listener's receiving apparatus works like a filter, rejecting ideas if they conflict with what she or he already believes. The listener may reject ideas by deliberately not hearing what is said, or by conscious decision—based either on fallacious judgment or rationalization to twist the meaning to fit preconceived ideas.

The environment or social setting involved in the communication affects the results. What might be accepted in private might easily be rejected if presented in public.

Overcoming Barriers

By watching the listener's expression and encouraging him to ask questions, barriers to communication may be removed. Wrongly interpreted messages may be corrected and clarified; the listener's subsequent behavior may give valuable clues as to the degree of understanding. Of course, feedback from written communications is not so easily obtained, but can best be judged by the action taken in relation to the communication.

Ten Commandments of Good Communication[4]

1   Seek to clarify your ideas before communicating.

2   Examine the true purpose of each communication.

3   Consider the total physical and human setting whenever you communicate.

4   Consult with others, where appropriate, in planning communications.

5   Be mindful, while you communicate, of the overtones as well as the basic content of your message.

6   Take the opportunity, when it arises, to convey something of help or value to the receiver.

7   Follow up your communications to make sure the message was understood.

8   Communicate for tomorrow as well as today.

9   Be sure your actions support your communications.

10   Seek not only to be understood but to understand—be a good listener.

CONCLUSION

All the knowledge in the world, all the skill possible, are meaningless without the vehicle of good interpersonal relations supported by a high level of communication. The thesis that energies previously (or currently) applied in maturation of a profession must be redirected, in part at least, toward reaching out to cooperate with others bears repeating. It is through cooperation and shared prestige that a profession expands its effectiveness, even while maintaining its separate identity and special contributions. Booker T. Washington's analogy sums this up succinctly: separate as the fingers, but united as the hand. That unity is in common objectives and coordination of effort because we understand one another. "While we hope that cooperation may be reduced to a science in time, we know that high levels of cooperation are already achievable by some professionals as an enviable talent and noble art."[1]

REFERENCES

1 Argyris, Chris, "Diagnosing Human Relations in Organizations: A Case Study of a Hospital," Yale University Labor and Management Center, New Haven, Conn., 1956.
2 Brown, Esther Lucile, "Newer Dimensions of Patient Care: Improving Staff Motivation and Competence in the General Hospital," Russell Sage Foundation, New York, 1962, pp. 81–101.
3 Collins, M. R., "Communication in Health Care," C. V. Mosby Company, St. Louis, 1977.
4 "Executive Communications," American Medical Association, n.d.,n. p.
5 Good, Paul, "The Individual," Time-Life Books, Chicago, 1974.
6 Hull, Calvin, and Gardner Lindzey, "Theories of Personality," John Wiley & Sons, Inc., New York, 1957.
7 Krech, David, R. S. Crutchfield, and E. L. Ballachey, "Individual in Society," McGraw-Hill Book Company, New York, 1962.
8 Murphy, Richard (ed.), "Status and Conformity," Time-Life Books, Chicago, 1976.
9 Steinberg, Rafael, "Man and the Organization," Time-Life Books, Chicago, 1975.
10 Wessen, A. F., Hospital Ideology and Communications between Ward Personnel, in E. G. Jaco (ed.), "Patients, Physicians, and Illness," The Free Press of Glencoe, New York, 1958, pp. 448–468.

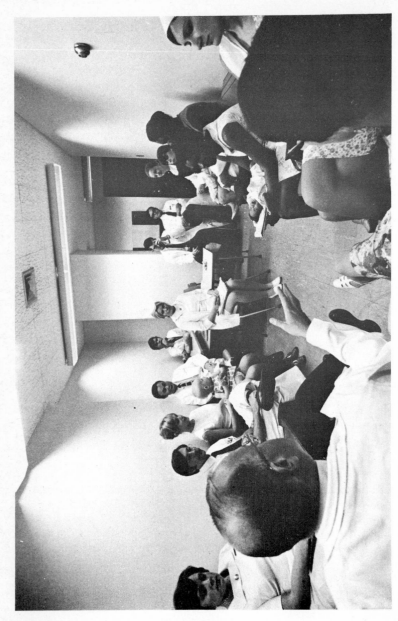

Group dynamics in action. (*Courtesy of Bill Rogers.*)

12
INTRODUCTION TO TEAM CONCEPTS

GENERAL CONSIDERATIONS

The "team" analogy has been used more generally in recent years, with application to any kind of group function. Its use in the health services context has come to the fore, particularly in response to criticism of the health care system, but also in response to the hopes of health professionals who seek to improve the quality of care they are providing. In some ways, the team analogy is counterproductive to the extent that a single leader is identified as the "captain," and that single leader is assumed to be the physician. This assumption follows the logic that the physician holds ultimate responsibility and authority. There are, however, many instances in which the physician may not be the *functional* member of the team in the hour-to-hour, or even day-to-day contacts with patients and their families.

Rather than using the athletic team as the model, and thus implying a definition of organizational structures and roles, a different model which allows for flexibility in organizational structure and definition of roles in relation to the patients' needs is preferable. Some have used the orchestra as the model, which more nearly approaches the desirable concept, but even here a defined leader is involved.

If one begins with a definition of the *health* team, there is more likelihood of promoting the flexibility that such a team must have to function maximally for the benefit of all concerned. Rubin, Plovnik, and Fry[23] have defined health team development as "learning and application of ways to manage interdependence." This is an apt phrase because it focuses on function rather than organizational structures. Managing interdependence is the critical element, challenging us to think through our attitudes and perceptions, the first of which is the proposition that no one, even the physician, is totally independent. All health professionals depend on colleagues and others from time to time in order for their services to be complete, yet this does not place them in subordinate positions that compromise their independence.

Whenever a task, or a cluster of tasks, requires the combined efforts of more than one person to complete, a team is involved. That team may be composed of as few as two members. In any case, managing interdependence well is critical to the outcome. This concept of a team applies to all situations that require group action, whatever the group may be labeled.

The need for health team development is the product of the complex character of the scientific, social, and economic aspects of health care. As noted earlier, the "knowledge explosion" and rapid rise of technological expertise and equipment has resulted in more and narrower specialization. Given the development of additional specialties and specialties within specialties, there is an accompanying increase in the numbers of health care personnel as well. This leads to intensification of the social forces of status-seeking, for example, which often negates the management of interdependence. The goal sought is independence, at least in the social sense. These scientific and social developments have had a profound, sometimes devastating effect on the economic aspects of health care. Costs have spiraled far above other costs of living, primarily because more personnel are required to perform the procedures involving more sophistication and more expensive equipment. The burden upon us is to find ways in which quality care can be delivered with more effectiveness and efficiency in the use of resources. The general consensus is that team development is a primary means by which this goal can be achieved. It is seen as a means by which a climate of support is built so that decision making by the group is facilitated and skills of individual members are put to their best uses.

COMPONENTS OF TEAM DEVELOPMENT AND IMPLEMENTATION

In Chapter 11, the discussion of groups and leaders was of a more general nature, applicable to a variety of situations. The focus now will be on those aspects that are critical to the functions of a team within the more limited context of health care delivery.

How Groups Develop

Tuckman's[28] developmental model provides a useful frame of reference in considering the changes that evolve as groups come together for task-oriented activities, find new goals to achieve, identify norms of behavior, and bring new members into the building process. Four stages have been defined by Tuckman: forming, storming, norming, and performing. In the forming stage, two characteristics are evident: testing and dependence. Each member of the group seeks first to determine the climate of the interpersonal behaviors that are expected, and, in task-oriented situations, to determine the dimensions of the work to be accomplished. This is the stage of becoming acquainted with people and functions. For the health team, this stage involves becoming familiar with what each of the members brings to the team in expertise (professional skills and knowledge) and personal attributes. These are then related to the roles and functions in the actual work of the team. The degree of dependence may differ according to the level of understanding of the group process, but frequently is manifested by a need to rely on externally established standards and readily identified leaders. Negotiations for the group's own standards and development of leaders from within the group may begin to occur as familiarity with one another and with the tasks takes shape.

The second stage, storming, can occur when members find expression of their own individuality to be the most important factor, and consequently they resist the formation of a team. Storming can develop into hostility and polarization, with the struggle typified by issues of control and conformity. When professional images or self-concepts are involved, this stage has even greater potential for a storm. As is common in any organization, agencies (such as hospitals) for health care are made up of many "vertical empires"—departments, and even sections within a department—that are instinctively self-protective and resistant to horizontal relationships. This characteristic reinforces the concept of individuality, stressing differences rather than similarities. Resolution of the conflict common to the storming stage comes with the realization that cooperation leads to gaining, rather than losing, position and individual value.

The third stage, norming, builds upon the resolution of conflict in establishing cooperation and trust. The group itself becomes important, and members seek to maintain the self-initiated standards and unique mission they have identified. Acceptance and valuing one another lead to cohesion that perpetuates the group, a primary function of norming.

Having formed, stormed, and normed, the group is ready for the fourth stage, performing. The group is now ready to function as a problem-solving unit that focuses on tasks, not persons, and seeks to use the capacity of each member to achieve success in its work. The structural and task aspects blend together so that there is unity in form and function.

These stages of group or team development are not necessarily discreet or time-related. Several may occur simultaneously, although as a rule, even in this situation, one stage predominates. The ease with which the development progresses from one to another is influenced significantly by the degree of trust and acceptance that exists.

LEADERSHIP

Having noted that leadership of the health team can and should shift among the members in relation to the tasks at hand, consideration of the styles of leadership or management each team member prefers or habitually uses is an important part of the process of becoming acquainted in the group. The Blake and Mouton[4] "Managerial Grid" instrument* is a valuable means of identifying leadership/management styles. This instrument is made up of five major categories dealing with functions, decision making, conflict with superiors or peers, conflict with subordinates, and creativity. In each category are five statements which are to be ranked on a scale of 1 to 5, least to most characteristic of oneself. The responses are scored and plotted on a grid, revealing the preferred style and the back-up styles which the individual will use in sequential order. Figure 12-1 shows the five major styles, plotting concern for people versus concern for task. Descriptions of these styles are based on extensive studies in management.

9/1: Leadership/management by Power: The task is *the* thing; decisions are made on the basis of the 9/1's official or unofficial power; the 9/1 cannot stand to lose; the 9/1 has little trust in

*Two films, "The Managerial Grid" featuring Blake and Mouton, are available from BNA Communications Inc., 9401 Decoverly Hall Road, Rockville, MD 20850.

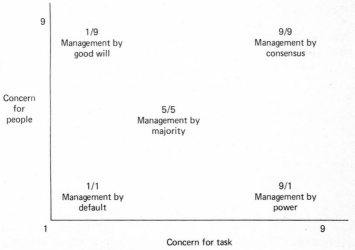

Figure 12-1 Styles of management.

Source: Adapted from R. R. Blake and J. Mouton, *The Management Grid*, Gulf Publishing Co., Houston, 1964, p. 10.

others' abilities to assume responsibility; control and direction are primary concerns of this leader.

1/9: Leadership/management by Goodwill: The 1/9 has high concern for people, but does not really trust the ability of others (or himself or herself) to deal with conflict, and so avoids it as much as possible; 1/9 focuses on maintaining, at least superficially, good interpersonal relations.

1/1: Leadership/management by Default: The 1/1 cares little about the task or people, and prefers not to make choices, resulting in inaction, avoidance, or withdrawal.

5/5: Leadership/management by Majority: Although the 5/5 is primarily concerned with the task, interpersonal issues will be given attention if they can lead to success with the task. Conflict is usually dealt with through negotiation and compromise. As a rule, the group's majority opinion dominates the decision making.

9/9: Leadership/management by Consensus: The 9/9 considers tasks and people as complementary, and emphasizes full participation by group members. Leadership functions may be shared by the 9/9.

There is a dynamic relationship between styles of leadership and the circumstances, as demonstrated by studies discussed by Carter and Shaw[6] who reported:

> When the situation is very favorable, the leader can be managing and controlling without arousing negative responses by group members; because things are going well, there is no reason to reject the directive behaviors of the leader. On the other hand, when the situation is highly unfavorable, things are going badly, and the group is in danger of falling apart, then directive leadership is required. . . . But if the situation is only moderately favorable, the group expects to be treated with consideration, and the permissive . . . leader is more effective.

Effective leadership calls for a repertoire of styles and the ability to respond to the demands of the situation by using the appropriate style. The circumstances will influence the shift from preferred to sequential back-up styles. For example, the preferred style may be 9/9, but when the group is found to be "talking the subject to death" a shift to 9/1 is indicated in order to make progress.

In addition to these circumstantial factors, the functions and characteristics of leadership are important components of the process. A leader focuses group behaviors, directs a group toward its goals, changes the level of the group's performance, and is generally selected by the group. These descriptions facilitate understanding how, in a smoothly functioning team, leadership may be shifted as necessary when accommodating the needs of the clientele of the team. For example, when the treatment plans should be focused on the rehabilitative activities of occupational therapy, the occupational therapist will be the leader, and others on the team will support those activities as they carry out their professional functions. The significant feature here is that the team members understand each other's roles and functions, and therefore are able to provide the necessary support.

ATTITUDES TOWARD TEAMWORK

In the discussion of the stages of group formation, trust was highlighted as a critical factor. For example, trust reflects attitudes of willingness to participate, and seeing the value of the other team members' contributions. This results in adaptibility, openness, and the cohesion of loyalty. Concerns are for one another rather than for oneself. Trust includes many of the positive attitudes that are implied by and inherent in the team itself.

Attitudinal changes occur relatively slowly, and are influenced by a variety of factors, as was pointed out in Chapter 11. Oftentimes, they may already be fully developed, and one has only to capitalize on them. This was demonstrated in pre- and postsurveys of attitudes of participants in a three-part workshop on team development* that covered a four-month period. These surveys demonstrated both stability of some attitudes and shifts in others, presumably because of learning during the workshop sessions. The following examples of stability and shifts after the program are of particular interest:

Both before and after the program, an equal number of participants preferred to work alone, but there was a shift from negative to positive in satisfaction with own job performance on the team. The participants perceived their job performance as being im-

*Conducted by the School of Associated Medical Sciences at the University of Illinois Medical Center in Chicago.

proved by team work, and after the program, more found it did not reduce performance.

After the program, 30 percent more of the participants found that input from coworkers facilitated the performance of their own tasks.

After the program, 70 percent perceived their work as not boring.

There was an increase of 30 percent in the number of participants who felt they were growing and developing in their work.

Fewer participants felt isolated in their work after the program.

30 percent more of the participants perceived themselves as team members after the program.

Both before and after the program, all the participants believed people can learn to work as a team.

In initiating a team-building program, one must be prepared for reluctance or resistance of varying degrees, and for the stages of group development to occur. Attitudes toward and perceptions of roles and functions are of critical importance, with perhaps the major task being translation of apprehensions of giving up status to assurances of gaining professional and personal satisfactions.

COMMUNICATION

As noted in Chapter 11, communication is the foundation upon which all social interaction is built, and poor communication is the proverbial foundation of sand. Becoming a team does not automatically invest members with communication skills. These must be honed by a conscious effort to improve on a continuing basis. Team efforts provide an excellent laboratory for practicing, obtaining feedback, and improving the ability to communicate.

VALUES

The process of valuing and the genesis of values have gradually become a major focus of attention. Consideration of values is a profitable study, for values are the determining factors in our personal and group processes of identification and ranking by priorities those in which we wish to make the heaviest investment. When we can focus on value development and clarification, the functions of enforcement and modeling fall into more appropriate uses.

Raths, Harmin and Simon[22] have identified seven criteria by which values may be processed. The authors make the point that values clarification is an important and continuous process, and urge its use in a conscious, reflective manner. The seven criteria to be used in values clarification proposed by these authors are:

Choosing freely: values must be freely selected if they are to be individually meaningful.

Choosing from among alternatives: obviously, choice means that there are alternatives, and in choosing, the valuing function operates.

Choosing after thoughtful consideration of the consequences of each alternative: This process furthers both weighing importance and understanding. Consideration of consequences furthers understanding of the implications inherent in the choice and commitment to the value.

Prizing and cherishing: A value is, by nature, a positive element, and the more it is esteemed and respected, the more functional it becomes.

Acting upon choices: To qualify as a value, there must be evidence that it has an effect on what and how one acts.

Repeating: Values persist in patterns of action, reappearing in different situations and at different times.

Values clarification using these criteria can be useful to the health team when formulating, implementing, and assessing achievement of objectives. When each team member can say that the group agrees that each of the criteria for a value has been met, they will have clarified the foundation upon which they are to function in relation to that value.

COMPONENTS OF TEAM FUNCTION

In the first module of their "Program for Health Team Development," Rubin, Plovnik and Fry[23] direct the learners' attention to the question of how they are doing as a team. The authors identify eight components of team function which they term "vital signs"— an analogy any health professional can readily understand. The eight components are

Goals (clarity and conflict)
Role ambiguity

Role conflict
Participation and influence
Commitment and understanding
Conflict management
Recognition and involvement
Support and cohesiveness

Note that these components or vital signs fall readily into the Tuckman developmental model of group development.

Setting goals and objectives is of primary importance in any task-oriented activity. "If you don't know where you're heading, how will you ever know when or if you've gotten there?" summarizes the importance of this aspect. A mission statement answers the question: what business are we really in. The next question, how do we operate, sets a philosophic context and clarifies the structure of relationships and communication. Typically, the team or group members will need to recognize their individual perceptions and values, and understand how they affect team goal setting, then agreement on objectives can be achieved. This is the clarification process, which facilitates resolution of goal conflicts, and helps the group identify priorities—putting values to work.

Role ambiguity is a common condition when any group begins to work together. In the health team development process, this calls for gaining understanding and appreciation of the expertise each has to offer, as well as individual styles of functioning. The question in this case is, how does who do what with and for whom. Considerable energy can be consumed, and tasks left undone when team members are unsure of the answer to this question.

Role conflict may be a product of role ambiguity to some extent, but it is more often a matter of jockeying for position. Resolution of role conflict is best achieved when there is understanding, accepting, and an appreciation of individuals in relation to the goals and objectives of the team. It calls for openness and genuine communication. In today's vernacular, "leveling with one another" expresses this aspect. Conflict arises when there are differing goals, differing means to a common goal, scarce goods (money, power, things, prestige, status), or threats to identity.

Active participation in team discussion brings about a greater sense of belonging as well as a higher level of understanding, resulting in productive decision making and implementation. Influence in decision making and implementation have the potential for negative behavior if the team members have not resolved ambiguities or negotiated what their roles will be in a given set of activities. The greater the sense of belonging and understanding, the more likely is there to be a positive influence that leads to individual and team satisfaction.

Commitment and understanding are natural partners, with minimal nonproductive energy consumption in resolving conflicts when each is at a high level. Again, communication that is open and genuine is vital.

Valuing is at the heart of recognition and involvement. When individual team members sense that their colleagues recognize and value what each has to contribute, involvement in the team's activities is a natural consequence.

Support and cohesiveness are evident when the team members pull together to get the job done. Pulling together means not only directing energies toward the same objectives, but appreciating good individual performance and assisting one another when problems arise. Again, personal and team satisfaction are at productive levels when there is team support and cohesiveness.

DECISION MAKING

All of life involves making decisions, every day, many times a day. Many times our decisions are made automatically, almost by reflex action. In productive teamwork, the same may be true of routine matters. When major decisions must be made that have long-range implications or consequences, that have an important influence on the team's individual and/or collective functions, or that involve choices that affect financial status (to name a few), the team must use a conscious approach. This involves first gathering as much information as possible about the problem (problem being used in the sense of something to be solved, not necessarily in the sense of something being wrong). Having the pieces of the puzzle—information—the next step is to explore the means to put them together, the means to solve the problem. Selection of the alternative that seems to have the most promise of effectiveness and efficiency is then made, followed by implementation and evaluation.

Hall, O'Leary, and Williams[14] have used the Blake-Mouton managerial grid to analyze five approaches to decision making, as shown in Figure 12-2. Four of the approaches to decision making involve power, conflict, manipulation, and numbers, all of which assume disparity between commitment and adequacy. The fifth assumes belief in consensus, which assumes that commitment and adequacy can be compatible.

9/1: Self-sufficient: Places adequacy above commitment, with quality uppermost. The base of operation is power.

1/9: Good neighbor: Accents commitment over adequacy, with goodwill uppermost. The base of operation is, in essence, fear of conflict.

1/1: Default: Neither commitment nor adequacy predominates. The base of operation is conformity and/or self-protection, e.g., if we don't go to bat we won't strike out. It does not recognize that no decision *is* a decision.

5/5: Traditional: Commitment and adequacy are equated. Trade-offs and compromises are common. The base of operation is in numbers (vote of the majority) and to some extent, manipulation.

9/9: Consensus: Assumes concern for both commitment and adequacy are complementary. With a high level of involvement, more alternative solutions are likely, and implementation has a greater chance of success because of the commitment that results from understanding and consensus.

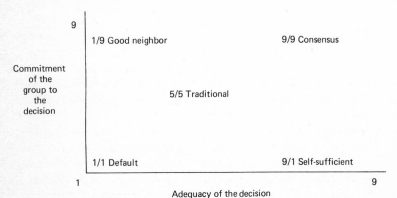

Figure 12-2   Decision-making grid.

Source: J. Hall, V. O'Leary and M. Williams, "The Decision-making Grid: A Model of Decision-making Styles." Cited in Bergquist et al. "Handbook for Faculty Development," Vol. 1, p. 158. Originally appeared in *California Management Review,* 1964.

SUMMARY

Health team development and implementation have become increasingly attractive in response to needed and desirable changes in health care delivery. While the discussion in this chapter has concentrated on health professionals, there are others to be recognized as team members, most certainly the patient, but also secretaries, receptionists, etc., who can and should be involved. Whenever possible, patient involvement in team efforts is advantageous. Any health professional can testify to the importance of the patient's cooperation and involvement in the diagnostic, therapeutic, and rehabilitative processes. With the attitude or operational set that the patient is the central imperative, and that team activities are oriented toward the tasks required in meeting the needs of patients, team development is accomplished with less stress.

Team development should accomplish at least four general goals in regard to the professional development of the individual. Stated behaviorally, these goals are that team members will:

Be knowledgeable about a wide range of health professionals' roles and functions, and value the legitimacy of each.

Be knowledgeable about various management styles and value the legitimacy of each.

Exchange ideas and expertise with colleagues and consultants about the team building/functioning processes.

Be able clearly and consistently to state and act upon their own personal and professional philosophies and values in the team concept.

Evaluation of the effectiveness of a health team may be made in terms of process and of product. There is greater ease in divising means to evaluate process because it is more easily defined conceptually and operationally. The "vital signs" scales recommended by Rubin, Plovnik, and Fry are examples of process evaluation. Product evaluation, on the other hand, is dependent on the specific health team goals established by the team itself. Saying that better health care delivery is the goal is not sufficient to evaluate product outcomes. Specific objectives that define precisely what the team means by better health care delivery are essential, and implies a knowledge of what the current status is. Quantitative product outcomes are, for example, an increase of numbers of patients served in a given time period without compromising services; reducing the time patients must spend waiting for services to be performed; reducing the incidence of repeat procedures because of error or omissions; reducing costs because of improved utilization of existing personnel, space, and equipment. A team may succeed well in the process, but its function in terms of product is the ultimate measure of success.

REFERENCES

1 Banta, H. D., and R. C. Fox, Role Strains of a Health Care Team in a Poverty Community, *Social Science and Medicine,* **6:**697–722, 1972.

2 Beckhard, Richard, Organizational Issues in the Team Delivery of Comprehensive Health Care, *Milbank Memorial Fund Quarterly,* July 1, 1972, pp. 287–316.

3 Bergquist, W. H., and S. R. Phillips, "A Handbook for Faculty Development," The Council for the Advancement of Small Colleges, in cooperation with Pacific Soundings Press, Cardiff-by-the-sea, Calif., vol. 1, 1975, vol. 2, 1977.

4 Blake, R. R., and Jane Mouton, "The Managerial Grid," Gulf Publishing Company, Houston, 1964.

5 Brill, Naomi, "Teamwork," J. B. Lippincott Company, Philadelphia, 1976.

6 Carter, L. F., et al., A Further Investigation of the Criteria for Leadership, in M. E. Shaw, "Group Dynamics: the Psychology of Small Group Behavior," McGraw-Hill Book Company, New York, 1971.

7 Cathcart, R. S., and L. A. Samovar, "Small Group Communication: A Reader," 2d ed., William C. Brown Company Publishers Dubuque, Iowa, 1970.

8 Collins, M. R., "Communication in Health Care," C. V. Mosby Company, St. Louis, 1977.

9 Eichhorn, Suzanne, "Becoming: The Evolution of Five Student Teams," Institute for Health Team Development, Bronx, N.Y., 1974.

10 Fast, Julius, "Body Language," M. Evans and Company, Inc., New York, 1970.

11 Films: "The Managerial Grid" and "The Grid Approach to Conflict Solving," BNA Communications Inc., Rockville, Md.

12 Good, Paul, "The Individual," Time-Life Books, Chicago, 1974.

13 Gurney, Wilma, The Social Worker's Responsibility in Interdisciplinary Treatment, *Tulane Studies in Social Welfare,* vol. 5, 1962, pp. 42–53.

14 Hall, J., V. O'Leary, and M. Williams, The Decision-making Grid: A Model of Decision-making Styles, *California Management Review,* **7:**43–54, 1964.

15 Kane, Rosalie A., The Interprofessional Team as a Small Group, *in* "Social Work in Health Care," vol. 1, Fall 1975.

16 Kindig, David A., Interdisciplinary Education for Primary Health Team Delivery: Perspectives in Primary Care Education, *J. Med. Ed.,* **50:**12, December 1975.

17 Leininger, Madeleine, About Interdisciplinary Health Education for the Future, *Nursing Outlook,* **19:**787–791, 1971.

18 Lekner, George, "Aids for Giving and Receiving Feedback," University of California at Los Angeles, n.d.

19 McDougall, M. G., and V. K. Elahi, The Comprehensive Health Care Project: A Multidisciplinary Learning Experience, *J. Med. Ed.,* **49:** 752–755, 1974.

20 Murphy, Richard (ed.), "Status and Conformity," Time-Life Books, Chicago, 1976.

21 Parker, Alberta W., "The Team Approach to Primary Health Care," University of California Extension, Berkeley, Calif., 1972.

22 Raths, L. E., M. Harmin, and S. B. Simon, "Values and Teaching," Charles E. Merrill Books, Inc. Columbus, Ohio, 1966, pp. 28, 29.

23 Rubin, I. M., M. S. Plovnik, and R. E. Fry, "Improving the Coordination of Care: A Program for Health Team Development," Ballinger Publishing Co., Boston, 1975.

24 Satir, Virginia, "Peoplemaking," Science and Behavior Books, Inc., Palo Alto, Calif., 1972.

25 Schmidt, Cheryl, Five Become a Team in Appalachia, *Am. J. Nsg.,* **75:**1314, 1315, 1975.

26 Shaw, M. E. (ed.), "Group Dynamics: The Psychology of Small Group Behavior," McGraw-Hill Book Company, New York, 1971, P. 277.

27 Steinberg, Rafael, "Man and the Organizations," Time-Life Books, Chicago, 1975.

28 Tuckman, Bruce W., Developmental Sequence in Small Groups, *Psych. Bull.,* **63:**384–399, 1965.

29 Weaver, Carl H., "Human Listening Process and Behavior," Bobbs-Merrill Series in Speech Communication, The Bobbs-Merrill Company, Inc., Indianapolis, 1972.

30 Willard, H. N. and S. V. Kasl, "Continuing Care in a Community Hospital," Harvard University Press, Cambridge, Mass. 1972.

31 Wise, Harold, The Primary Care Health Team, *Arch. Int. Med.,* **130:** 438–444, September 1972.

32 Wise, Harold, R. Beckhard, I. Rubin, and A. Kyle, "Making Health Team Work," Ballinger Publishing Co., Boston, 1974.

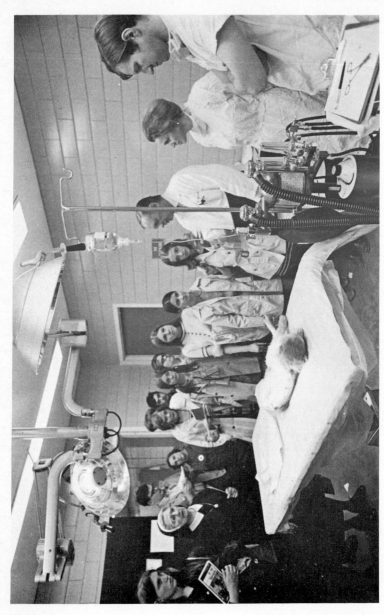

The chief of surgery explains research using animals. *(Courtesy of Bill Rogers.)*

13
INTRODUCTION TO RESEARCH

In the twentieth century, research is vital to almost every activity—from cooking dinner to exploring outer space—and the researcher is regarded as one of society's elite. Others may be somewhat awed by the researcher, whose activities take on a certain aura of glamour. Many college students look forward to the world of research as their life's work. Often, the attitudes of "ordinary" persons may prevent them from thinking that they could possibly do research or contribute to that being done by others. True, research does require depth of knowledge and facility with techniques, but any professional worker, especially in the health care field, can make significant contributions, or ask pertinent questions that can lead to valuable research. An open mind, curiosity, a habit of noting subtle variations of standard techniques—these are the researcher's basic attributes.

DEFINITIONS

Research is essentially a problem-solving process, a systematic, intensive study directed toward fuller scientific knowledge of the subject studied. In solving problems, research answers questions.

There are two common divisions, or kinds, of research—basic and applied. In basic research, the goal is knowledge for the sake of knowledge. Applied research is practical, in that it attempts to find the means of using knowledge. Research is extended by development—the conversion of knowledge into useful tools.

Both basic and applied research have three levels of investigation: exploratory, descriptive, and experimental. *Exploratory research* investigates the important variables in a given situation. *Descriptive research* asks how these variables are related to one another. *Experimental research* concerns itself with the effects of the variables upon one another.

As a problem-solving process, the steps in research are to:

1 Identify, limit, and define the problem
2 Identify basic assumptions
3 Recognize and assemble relevant facts and principles
4 Arrange assumptions, premises, and conclusions
5 Select a reasonable plan of action
6 Act in accord with the plan
7 Evaluate the outcome

USES OF HYPOTHESES AND THEORIES
Hypotheses

A hypothesis is a statement of relationships between variables. Its function is to link generalized theory to facts, to guide research design, and to determine what is to be measured. *Predictive hypotheses* are commonly framed as "If . . . then . . ." statements. Operational hypotheses include some explanation of, or rationale for the prediction. If the prediction is confirmed by research, not only is a relationship among the variables confirmed, but the explanatory principles are also confirmed. An example of this type of hypothesis is the social psychologists' theory that people will be aggressive when some of their needs are frustrated. Such a hypothesis could be stated, "Because certain needs are being frustrated in the people living in area X, there will be demonstrations of protest." *Curiosity-testing hypotheses* stem from questions such as "I wonder what the relationship is between variable X and variable Y?"

Variables are those elements involved in an event or process that (1) are changed, or (2) cause change. The variable that is subject to alteration by the introduction of a given factor (as well as the intensity of that factor) is termed the *affect,* or *dependent* variable. If heat is used as an example of such a factor, it is obvious that heat itself causes change, and the degree of heat (intensity) influences the degree of change. The variable that causes change is termed the *causal,* or *independent* variable. In the example cited, heat is the independent variable, and is the one that can be manipulated to determine its effect on the dependent variable. The experimenter has control over the independent variable, and observes changes in the dependent variable.

Theories

A theory is like a map on which a few points are charted, leaving the road between them to be inferred. A well-outlined map can be filled in as more details are learned; a poor map should be discarded, for it can lead one astray. A good theory is comprehensive and explicit, and generates useful research. A good theory may lead to previously overlooked relationships. For example, the germ theory pointed out relationships that had long been present in fact, but made no sense until a theory was formulated relating one fact to another, and making it possible to test the theory's reliability.

Theories focus attention on relevant data by stating what to look for and how to describe it. Theories anticipate laws, just as laws predict events. Newton's theory of attraction of bodies to the earth led to the law of gravity. Scientific laws cannot be "broken" as legal rules can be. The drunk who proclaimed that he was going to break the law of gravity discovered, when he attempted to do so, that he was merely demonstrating it.

The basis of a theory may be personal, historical, sociologic (cultural), or philosophic. The *personal* basis determines the researcher's interests and reveals what he is influenced by, or believes in. A prime example is given by Galileo's absorption in the study of astronomy and the physics of motion mechanics. In addition, Galileo's strong beliefs were counter to those of his time. *Historical* bases provide the foundation upon which others work. For example, Becquerel's studies of radioactivity in uranium were essential to Pierre and Marie Curie, enabling them to continue working with pitchblende until they discovered the element radium. *Sociologic,* or cultural, bases can influence progress in research. Greek thinkers were strongly affected by class distinctions that proscribed work by the elite, and were uninterested in doing the work necessary to test their theories. The quality and state of the development of the researchers' society shape their choice of subjects and the available facilities, and supply the basis of the knowledge that they might work with in developing their theories. *Philosophic* bases also affect the fruitfulness of research. As demonstrated in the Middle Ages, little progress can be made when political and religious leaders suppress freedom to question and make discoveries. With the new freedoms of the eighteenth and nineteenth centuries, thinkers and researchers were freed from stereotypes and began to work creatively.

Many scientific theories and laws are developed from data obtained by observation alone. Certain objects of scientific study, such as stars, can be observed, but cannot be subjected to purposeful changes, by the experimenter. Experimental investigation is essentially purposeful. It consists of so changing the conditions of observation that errors are minimized as much as possible, and the data obtained by observation point to an answer to the question posed by the experimenter.

Simple observations have sometimes led to ridiculous errors, and it is well to be wary of this method. For example, until 1668, it was commonly believed that a piece of decaying meat turned into worms and flies. This belief was the result of observation alone and the basis of the theory of spontaneous generation (heterogenesis), which stated that the dead tissues of animals could come to life in the form of worms or insects. The fact that a living fly might have deposited eggs on the meat was not considered. This is an example of an environmental error, a failure to recognize something in the surroundings that could alter the outcome. Francesco Redi challenged this theory by exposing fresh pieces of meat to the heat of July, but protected the meat from flies by sealing it in a glass flask, or closing the mouth of the flask with a fine Naples veil. The meat decayed, but no worms or flies were generated. Other pieces of meat, left in open flasks, were soon infested. Redi's was one of the earliest examples of experimental control.

WHY RESEARCH?

Once considered suspect, now a glamorous pursuit, research makes a number of valuable contributions. Research is widely used to:

1 Discover new facts about known phenomena
2 Find answers to problems that are only partially solved by existing methods and information
3 Improve existing techniques and develop new instruments or products
4 Discover previously unrecognized substances or elements
5 Discover pathways of action of known substances and elements

Success in research depends greatly on instruments and techniques with which to probe the unknown. Certain research problems cannot be approached without first devising specific instruments. The space exploration programs demonstrate this principle, and as a consequence of developments for this program, other areas of research benefit. Certainly the instruments used to monitor the astronauts' physical responses to space flight have valuable applications for the earthbound—and other benefits will undoubtedly be investigated.

Early in what is now called the new scientific age, each branch of science worked independently and conducted its own investigations. However, now that many of the sciences have gone beyond the gross areas of discovery, many specialties must pool their efforts to focus on certain problems.

ISSUES IN BIOMEDICAL RESEARCH

With the discovery of the structure of deoxynucleic acid (DNA), which is the foundation of genetic mechanisms, followed by research studies and technology that make possible the "slicing" of the DNA molecule and the inserting of specific genes (recombinant DNA), a whole new era was ushered in. Recognizing the potential for "genetic engineering" to produce powerful strains of pathogenic bacteria for example, the scientists involved in the research voluntarily called a moratorium, and in a conference at Asilomar, developed the first set of guidelines for such research. Recombinant DNA research has become a cause célèbre, due to its profound implications as a major scientific breakthrough. One consequence has been the involvement of both the legislative and regulatory bodies of the federal government, and, in some cases, local governments.[9] The National Institutes of Health has developed guidelines backed with the authority of governmental regulations. Several bills have been introduced in Congress dealing with recombinant DNA. Senator Edward Kennedy, speaking to the Medical Writers Association in late 1977, affirmed the importance of public as well as scientific participation in the processes of "evaluation, development and implementation of our national policy toward science and medical research." The issues attendant to recombinant DNA research will undoubtedly continue to engage the public in science as has no previous scientific discovery in the "nature and extent of regulation necessary, definitions of activities to be regulated, penalties for noncompliance, and state and local preemption."[9] Senator Adlai Stevenson called for Congress to "enact legislation which is essentially interim in character and which permits great flexibility in accommodating to the scientific evidence as it is developed."[17]

Another important issue is that of NIH assessing technology, as exemplified by the controversy over methods used to detect mammary cancer at an early stage of its development. The question in this case is whether or not mammography (a radiologic screening procedure) may precipitate the development of as many breast tumors as it detects.[5] In addition to this extremely important facet, consideration must also be given to the problem of proceeding with mastectomy on the basis of the radiologic diagnosis. For example, on the basis of tissue examination, 66 out of 1,850 women diagnosed as having cancer did not, yet many had had radical mastectomies. Again, a broader base of input has been used in addressing the issue of screening mammography. NIH called upon the expertise of ethicists, economists, physicians, and researchers whose work did not involve breast cancer, or the point of view of women, in order to review the mammography program. The three-day session, which included testimony from many individuals and organizations, resulted in recommended guidelines for the screening program.

Clinical trials as a research activity are also coming under scrutiny, especially where terms of informed consent of the subjects and discontinuance of participation are involved. Methodology is being looked at particularly in terms of the time and expense involved and numbers of participants required. These determine how cost-effective the study may be, especially when the clinical trials focus on preventive measures such as diet patterns and reduction of blood cholesterol levels.[3]

RESPONSIBILITIES IN MEDICAL RESEARCH

Any researcher making investigations in the field of medicine has a responsibility to society that is potentially greater than the physician's in his or her comparatively limited physician-patient relationship. What the researcher discovers might have implications for all mankind. As one famous Nobel prize winner has said, "From my own experience, I do not know of any scientific or technical advance of importance that did not make utterly unexpected demands on knowledge from unpredictable sources."[*] These matters, and others as well, are addressed by Eisenberg[6] in his article on the relationship of society's needs and medical research.

It sometimes happens that a researcher's discoveries generate false hopes for a panacea or, at least, for a cure for a given disease. For this reason, as well as for scientific validity, expectations for the new discovery must be tempered by experience. Such experience may be gained by extensive field trials such as those for vaccines that help control disease incidence, or additional intensive studies of the relationships of newly identified etiologic agents such as those of a virus, which appears to be associated with specific types of cancer.

In the case of a field trial, the process is one of using the vaccine on a appropriate sample of the population. The first step is to determine whether or not the subjects have any specific antibod-

---

[*]Quoted by Joshua Lederberg, Some Problems of Instant Medicine, *Saturday Review,* May 6, 1967, p. 70.

ies before the vaccine is administered; the second is to test for the antibody response after receiving the vaccine. Finally, statistical analysis must be made of disease incidence in the general population, as compared to the sample in the field test. With these data, conclusions about the efficacy, safety, and acceptability of the new vaccine can be drawn.

The ubiquitous problem of cancer—etiologic agent(s), prevention, early diagnosis, and reliable cures—engages the thought and energies of many researchers. Because of the character of cancer and its high incidence as a cause of death, cancer research programs are given high priority in federal funding support. There is growing evidence implicating viruses as etiologic agents of some types of cancer, supported by known instances in animals. Obviously, since one would not risk inducing such a disease in human subjects, it is necessary to study those who have the disease "naturally" by isolating the same virus from many tumors and making statistical comparisons between the incidence of the presence of the virus and the incidence of the disease. A current example of this simplified description of a complex process is that of a herpes virus apparently associated with cancer in the female genital tract. Similar intensive studies are required in research focused on prevention and cure like that being conducted by immunologists.

The "fall-out" from research on diseases can have sociological and economic, as well as medical impact, especially when premature decisions are made on the basis of insufficient data. One example of this is seen in the rash of state laws requiring the testing of newborns for phenylketonuria. This is a condition that results from an inborn error of metabolism, and can result in mental retardation if untreated at the early stages. With the laudable intent of preventing mental retardation by early diagnosis and proper treatment, some state laws require the test on all newborns. When these laws were first implemented, it was found that PKU occurred in about 1 in 15,000 births. Problems have arisen because false-positive results (pseudo-PKU) and too vigorous treatment of the disease have their own deleterious results.

Another example of "fall-out" effects of research discoveries involves sickle-cell anemia. Linus Pauling opened the door to accurate diagnosis of diseases involving molecular aberrations when he found that the hemoglobin molecule of sickle-cell anemia patients was of a different amino-acid construction from that of normal hemoglobin. More reliable tests for S-hemoglobin are now available, and it is possible to identify the "trait" (a combination of S and A hemoglobin genes without manifested disease), and the disease (SS gene combination). Misunderstanding the differences between trait and disease has resulted in economic hardships such as the denial of certain kinds of employment, or high insurance premiums. Sociologically, the impact of knowledge generated by research is felt in marriage and in birth control. If the prospective bride and groom each have the trait, there is a 1:4 possibility that their offspring will inherit the S gene from each parent and thus have the disease. Can their expectations of a normal family relationship be denied by the risk involved? Such a question can only be answered by the individuals concerned, after accurate genetic counseling. Screening for sickle-cell disease must be accompanied by genetic counseling in order to reduce fears and suggest appropriate birth-control practices.

Sickle-cell disease research has also had political implications. Since the incidence of the disease is highest among the black population, some political leaders have made the accusation that an intended genocide is the reason research on prevention and cure has not been as vigorous or fully funded as other specific research projects. With the 1972 federal support appropriated specifically for the study of this disease, and with campaigns for donations to nonprofit organizations advancing in the same purpose, the argument now has no apparent validity. It is much more reasonable to assume that, even though a great deal of research was being conducted during the years since Pauling's discovery, that research did not receive as much publicity, or perhaps was not treated with as great a sense of urgency as research into other areas.

ETHICS IN MEDICAL RESEARCH

The value of human life must be uppermost in the mind of the bona fide medical researcher. This belief assumes respect to persons, and for their rights and privileges, which include the right to protection from harm. In recognition that such an assumption must have the support of guidelines and/or regulations, a growing body of formal and legal documents has been developed as a result of the Nuremberg trials to legislate regulations and guidelines for research involving human subjects.

In clinical investigation, subjects are selected, not accepted, as they are when patients consult the physician. This selection of subjects involves important ethical considerations that are not always neatly defined. For example, when the subjects, such as students or prisoners, are under the additional pressure of possible gain for participating in research, are they in fact volunteers? The Secretary of DHEW has ruled that, for federally sponsored or funded research, prisoners may not be used as subjects when there are serious hazards involved. The current concern for protection of subjects reveals the increased sensitivity to individual rights in general. An extreme case in point is the long-term study of the effects of untreated syphilis that was begun in 1932 by the Public Health Service venereal disease section.[1] At that time, 625 black men, mostly poor and uneducated, were selected, of whom 425 had latent syphilis. The 200 who did not have the disease were the control group. The incentives for participating in the study were free treatment for other illnesses, free hot lunches, and free burial after autopsy had been performed. The study was continued even after the discovery of penicillin, the treatment of choice for syphilis. Not until 1972, when an alert news investigator noted and reported that withholding treatment from the 74 surviving subjects was intentional, did the study come to the attention of the public. An investigation was ordered in response to this "moral and ethical nightmare," as it was termed by Senator William Proxmire. But not much could be expected of the probe, for the damage was long since done and those responsible were gone.

Selection of subjects in this manner should be impossible to duplicate now that there are regulations covering protection of research subjects, not only from harm, but in their rights of privacy as well. At the national level, the NIH Office for Protection of Research Risks is responsible for monitoring implementation of the regulations. Penalties for noncompliance include fines as well as loss of funding. Informed consent of the subjects is an absolute requirement.

All institutions conducting biomedical research are required to have committees or a board which review proposals for compliance with ethical and legal standards, and which monitor approved projects during the research process. The director for a research project must provide evidence that the proposed methods either do not involve human subjects, or if they do that (1) the potential for harm is minimal, (2) the procedure for obtaining informed consent is acceptable, and (3) there is a means of treatment, should the subject sustain injury.

RESEARCH METHODOLOGY
Processes of Research

Research is systematic study, following a set of rules or procedures. The so-called scientific method is such a set of procedures built sequentially:

1 Observation: An unsystematic, introductory process in which one becomes acquainted with the variables.
2 Description: A beginning systematic process in which the variables are separated from context and described, such as groupings of similar things or events.
3 Measurement: Description becomes more sophisticated and useful at this step because of quantification in numbers, size, and intensity.
4 Evaluation: Acceptance or rejection of information obtained from the measures of variables.

These procedures lead to the formation of theories and principles:

1 Induction: A synthesis of general principles and findings; going from the general to the specific
2 Deduction: Arriving at a principle or theory from the evidence supplied by the findings; going from the specific to the general
3 Explanation of the events or findings in the light of theory

Following this initial formulation of theory, hypotheses are developed and tested to refine the theory. After testing these hypotheses, the researcher proceeds with the following steps:

1 Correction: Using the results from deduction and testing, the refinements subsequent to increased knowledge or information are fed back into the theory.

2 Reduction: Excess verbiage is trimmed, and basic assumptions are further generalized and reduced in number.

Form of Reporting Research

Reports of research generally follow a pattern made up of a number of sections, the organization of which aids in judging the quality of the research. These sections are, in order of appearance:

1 Purpose: a statement of the topic

2 Hypothesis: what question is to be answered by the research

3 Review of the related literature: what others have done

4 Methodology: the procedure used, stating choices of subjects or materials tested; how and why they were chosen; the application of the dependent variable; steps used in the tests; statistical tests used to determine the levels of significance

5 Results: tables, graphs, etc., to present data concisely

6 Discussion: the results obtained in the light of theoretical application

7 Conclusion: results from the test of the hypothesis

8 Recommendations: further studies, if indicated

Abstracts

A *descriptive abstract,* sometimes called an indicative or alerting abstract, presents in general terms what the article is about, but doesn't reveal the actual observations and conclusions. It merely alerts the reader, who must read the original to get the facts. Descriptive abstracts are useful for survey articles and review articles or for extended discussions too long or too detailed to justify a fuller abstract.

An *informative abstract,* also called an *informational abstract,* is a comprehensive summary of the observations and conclusions of the original article. Standing alone, it informs the reader.

An *extract,* like an abstract, summarizes, but does so by quoting important sentences from the original rather than by paraphrasing. Quotations may be selected by a human analyst or a machine.

Telegraphic abstracts are detailed indexes composed of significant words selected from a document and stored on coded tape. The reels of tape contain all the information of a conventional card datalogue or index, and also supply the main content of the articles. Translated into computer code, the information can be electromagnetically retrieved and translated into a comprehensive survey.

RESEARCH EVALUATION OUTLINE

In order to have some criteria for judging the reliability and validity of test results, and to test one's own research design and results, it is helpful to ask pertinent questions about the problems, designs, sampling, controls, measurements, treatment of data, results, and conclusions of the author of the report.

Problem

1 Is the problem stated clearly?

2 Does the problem have a solution the way it is formulated?

3 Is it clear whether this is a normative, or survey study or a study to test a hypothesis?

4 Is the literature of previous studies of the same or related problems adequately reviewed or taken into account?

5 Are the essential concepts necessary to understanding the problem defined?

6 Is the context of the problem described so that what is included and excluded is readily apparent?

7 Is the seriousness or importance of the problem sufficiently developed so that judgment can be made about the suitability of the methods?

8 Are the consequences of the possible findings pointed out?

Design

1 Was the design of the study planned and evaluated beforehand?

2 Does the design take into account all the pertinent aspects of the study: subjects and materials; environments; manipulated variables; measurements and observations; statistical methods?

3 Is the design succinctly presented so that it can be readily understood?

4 Were alternative designs considered and reasons for their rejection given?

5   Are the compromises made with an ideal design described?
6   Is it possible for the design to answer the questions posed?
7   Can the design efficiently solve the problems in terms of money, subjects, and time?

Sampling of Subjects or Materials
1   Is the sample adequately described?
2   Of what population is the sample representative?
3   Is the sample an appropriate one for the purposes of the study?
4   Were the subjects selected according to the design of the study and with regard to the statistical methods to be used?
5   Is the size of the sample adequate?
6   Was the sample collected for the purposes of this study or for other purposes?
7   Are the methods of sampling described?

Controls
1   What controls were exercised through sampling?
2   What controls were exercised by selection of settings? By natural habitat?
3   What controls were exercised by experimental manipulation?
4   Were the conditions the same for all subjects or were adjustments made?
5   If controls were changed, were results analyzed with respect to the altered conditions?
6   Are there any important controls missing from the study?
7   Were the usual controls for a study of this type absent, and if so, was the absence justified?
8   Could any additional controls have been included that would have increased the efficiency of the study?

Measurements
1   Are the techniques of measurement adequately described?
2   From the information presented, could the measurements be repeated by another investigator?
3   Are the measurements suitable for the problem?

Data Treatment
1   Are the methods of recording and the treatment of data described?

2　Are the statistical procedures described and are they suitable?

3　Are the significant tests described and are they suitable?

Results

1　Are the results or data adequately presented so the reader may verify the author's statements about them?

2　Are estimates of error provided?

3　Have the essential relationships posed by the problem been analyzed and tested for significance?

4　Are the results clearly reported in tables and graphs so that others may use the data or reproduce the results?

Conclusions

1　Does the author draw conclusions about the major problem of the study?

2　Are the conclusions clearly supported by the data?

3　Are important reservations or qualifications pointed out?

4　Are artifacts or spurious relations pointed out?

5　Has the author overlooked important aspects of the results?

6　Are necessary modifications of theory, current interpretations of data or practice pointed out?

7　Are the results interpreted in relation to other published information and is their significance for related fields pointed out?

8　Are the methods used in the study critically reviewed in the light of the obtained results?

9　Are the interpretations, implication for future research, and development of new methods appropriate for the present study, or do they reflect an overestimation or underestimation of the significance of the study?

REFERENCES

1　A Matter of Morality, *Time,* Aug. 7, 1972, p. 54.

2　Barber, Bernard, et al., "Problems of Social Control in Medical Experimentation," Russell Sage Foundation, New York, 1973.

3　Clinical Trials: Methods and Ethics Are Debated, *Science,* **198:**1127–1129, Dec. 16, 1977.

4　Culliton, Barbara, Genetic Screening: States May be Writing the Wrong Kind of Laws, *Science,* **191:**926–929, May 5, 1976.

5　Culliton, Barbara, Mammography Controversy: NIH's Entreé into Evaluating Technology, *Science,* **198:**171–173, Oct. 14, 1977.

6   Eisenberg, Leon, The Social Imperatives of Medical Research, *Science,* **198:**1105–1110, Dec. 16, 1977.

7   Goodfield, June, Humanity in Science: A Perspective and a Plea, *Science,* **198:**580–585, Nov. 11, 1977.

8   Goodfield, June, "Playing God: Genetic Engineering and the Manipulation of Life," Random House, New York, 1977.

9   Halvorsen, H. O., Recombinant DNA Legislation—What Next? *Science,* **198:**357, Oct. 28, 1977.

10 Hook, Lucyle, and Mary Gaver, "The Research Paper," 3d ed., Prentice-Hall, Inc., Englewood Cliffs, N.J., 1962.

11 How to Present a Scientific Paper, *Therapeutic Notes,* Feb. 10, 1963, publication of Parke Davis & Co., Detroit, Mich.

12 Medical Research: Statistics and Ethics. A collection of papers presented at the Birnbaum Memorial Symposium. *Science,* **198:**677–699, Nov. 18, 1977.

13 Price, Derek, Ethics of Scientific Publication, *Science,* **144:**655–657, May 8, 1964.

14 Rogers, Michael, "Biohazard," Alfred A. Knopf Inc., New York, 1977.

15 Roth, Russell, The Dilemmas of Human Experimentation, *Modern Medicine,* **43:**56–61, February 1975.

16 Shapley, Deborah, Research Management Scandals Provoke Queries in Washington. *Science,* **198:**804–806, Nov. 25, 1977.

17 Stevenson, Adlai, Remarks to the Senate, *Congressional Record,* Sept. 22, 1977.

18 Veatch, R. M., Human Experimentation: The Crucial Choices Ahead, *Prism,* **2:**58–61, July 1974.

19 Visscher, M. B., Moral Values vs Scientific Progress, *Modern Medicine,* **43:**62–64, February 1975.

20 Wade, Nicholas, "The Ultimate Experiment: Man-made Evolution," Walker & Co., New York, 1977.

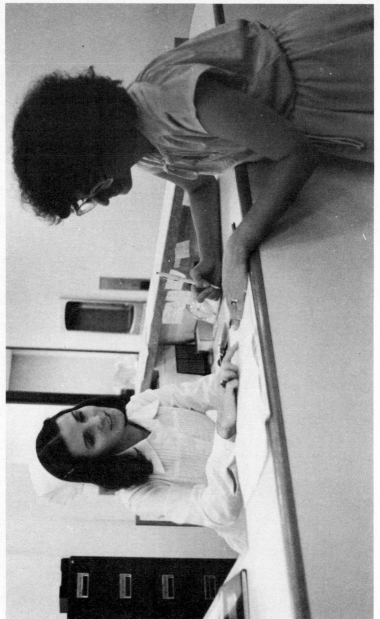

Every staff member can help patients by careful use of resources. *(Photo courtesy of Milton Heiberg.)*

14

INTRODUCTION TO FINANCIAL ASPECTS OF HEALTH CARE

GENERAL CONSIDERATIONS

The truism that "there are no free lunches" is especially applicable to concerns in health care, for costs must be paid by public funds (taxes), insurance (employers, individuals), or the individual. Cost of health care is the pivotal factor in determining access to, quality, and utilization of the wide range of services available. Economic considerations often are important determinants of the choice of careers and sites of employment, and thus influence both the numbers and distribution of health care manpower. They are also determinants of what kinds of services are or can be offered that involve specific kinds of equipment and especially expert personnel.

Accountability for expenditures is a particular responsibility of government, third-party payers, and physicians, each seeking to influence decisions on health care, and is of great concern to the patient. Governmental entities are accountable because they must show a balance between expenditures and the benefits to society on whose behalf tax dollars are used. The magnitude of this is revealed in the fact that in 1975, Medicare was the source of payment for 40 percent of hospital costs. Third-party payers are accountable because they must maintain a balance between income from premiums and expenditures lest they become insolvent, and of course, they are also interested in making a profit. Physicians are accountable because they hold the key to what goods and services are used by the patient: they prescribe drugs, order diagnostic and therapeutic services, and determine admission to and discharge from institutional care. The patient is naturally concerned because of the impact of the cost on the individual pocketbook, yet the patient does not have the "luxury" of deciding the what, when, and how of care as a buyer.

In the United States, the pattern of spiraling costs of health care is clearly shown in a comparison of figures for 1960 and 1975.

Year	Total expenditure	Per capita expenditure	% of gross national product
1960	$ 25.9 billion	$141	5.2
1975	118.5 billion	547	8.3

The factors feeding this marked increase of expenditures are formed in a complex of burgeoning medical technologies, specialization, increased utilization, increased numbers of personnel required, increases in minimum wages, increased paperwork dealing with insurance forms and governmental documents, and inflation. Efforts toward cost containment are directed at improvements in cost-effectiveness—"more bang for the buck," to put it in the vernacular. Cost-effectiveness applies not only to the obvious factors but to the administrative costs as well.

Imposition of seemingly arbitrary cost-containment measures is sure to rouse protests from nearly every sector of the health care industry. The issues become the determination of acceptable levels of access, quality, and cost, then the acceptable balance among these factors. Having made these determinations, subsequent plans for achieving the best payoff for the dollars available are more likely to lead to cost containment. Modification of educational programs could result as well. For example, medical education does not include consideration of the cost of services to the patient. One wonders what might happen if medical students were taught to weigh economic as well as medical considerations in their selection of the goods and services they order for their patients. What if the charges for the goods and services were included on the requisition forms? Would the physician think twice about ordering something that is "interesting but not necessary"? Would standing orders be monitored more carefully so that they are discontinued, rather than allowed to go on and on?

The physician is not alone in accountability, of course. Every health professional must be careful in performing services for patients, not only in terms of quality per se, but in order to avoid economic consequences of error. For example, when having to repeat a diagnostic procedure means the patient's stay in the institution is even one day longer than necessary, it would involve an additional day's room charge—as much as $200, perhaps more. Cost containment is *everyone's* business and responsibility.

FINANCING HEALTH CARE

There are six general categories of methods to finance health care: personal, charitable, industrial, voluntary insurance plans, social insurance plans, and use of governmental general revenue funds. Combinations of these methods are common.

Personal payment usually applies to ambulatory care, dental care, and drugs.

Charitable support for health care is declining except for that provided by voluntary agencies such as the American Cancer Society. Even in these cases, the support tends to be minor, covering loan of equipment, transportation for office visits, and the like.

Industrial support for health care may be that which is provided on the premises of the company or institution. Many industrial companies maintain a health service for employees, but the services are for preventive medicine and/or work-related injuries. As noted earlier, the railroad industry was a pioneer in providing employees medical services, some having a hospital system as well. In addition, there are some group health maintenance organization plans such as the Kaiser-Permanente model which offer comprehensive care.

Voluntary insurance plans are offered by a wide range of insurance companies, all of which require premium payments for specified types and amounts of benefits. The voluntary plans may be for the individual or for groups, the latter being less expensive. Basic group plans are frequently provided by employers, with the employee paying the difference in premiums for additional types and amounts of coverage. Health care insurance is one of the important fringe benefits sought and maintained in labor union contracts.

Voluntary insurance plans may be contracts with a medical service group on an annual per capita fee basis, or on a fee-for-service basis. An interesting comparison was made by Anderson and Sheatsly[1] in New York City. The Health Insurance Plan of Greater New York (HIP) contracted with medical groups using an annual capitation prepayment that covered all services for enrollees, using 30 medical groups. Group Health Insurance, Inc. (GHI) contracted with individual physicians on a fee-for-service basis. More GHI enrollees (11 percent) than HIP enrollees (6.3 percent) were hospitalized, and GHI patients had longer hospital stays as well as a higher incidence of surgical procedures. The number of physician visits was about the same for both groups.

Social insurance includes Medicare, Medicaid, and Workmen's Compensation programs. These are mandatory programs established by law, and are, in effect, a form of taxation. *Medicare* is the federal program administered under the Social Security Administration for persons over 65 and other recipients of Social Security benefits. When hospitalized, the individual pays $144 and Medicare pays the balance for 60 days. For the next 30 days, the individual pays $36 per day and Medicare pays the balance. Nursing home care is covered for at least 100 days following hospitalization. Coverage for doctor's services is available through a monthly premium of $7.70, the benefits being as much as 80 percent of the costs beyond the first $60 per year. Other services covered are home health visits, diagnostic tests, and ambulance service.

Medicaid programs are combinations of federal and state funding administered by the state. The ratio of federal to state funding varies from 50 percent to 83 percent, depending on the state's economic status. Medicaid provides assistance to welfare recipients and other poor as defined by elibigility requirements. Benefits are for goods and services.

Workmen's Compensation plans are at the state level, covering work-related injury or illness. Employers pay the state at prescribed levels for each employee.

In the United States, *general revenue* funds support public health service programs. In other countries such as England, Sweden, West Germany, and Russia, all health care goods and services benefits are paid from general revenues. Among the issues debated in relation to national health insurance in the United States is the question of the use of general revenue sources rather than specified sources such as the current Medicare-Social Security Administration.

The American Medical Association set up a National Commission on the Cost of Medical Care which began work in March 1976. The charge to the Commission was to:

Describe the health care delivery system
Identify the factors underlying the rising costs of medical care
Review and evaluate existing research on the causes of medical care cost inflation
Evaluate the impact of pending or future health care programs on the health care delivery system and medical care costs
Recommend policies that will contribute to containment of medical expenditures while providing quality of care to the public
Recommend direction for future research programs, including detailed description of existing data bases

Obviously, the Commission's tasks are formidable and, if accomplished at all, should make highly significant contributions to understanding the problems of financing health care and pointing toward their resolutions. As the experience in Canada has shown, the development of a successful national health insurance program needs the cooperation of those who render services, and those who organize and administer the program; to proceed without a solid base of cooperation, one courts disaster.[2]

NATIONAL HEALTH INSURANCE

Since 1974, more than 12 bills have been drafted for a variety of types of National Health Insurance (NHI). They may be classified

Table 14-1 Proposals for National Health Insurance

| Proposal | Funding | Coverage | | Private carrier involvement | Federal contract with providers |
		Catastrophic only	Comprehensive		
Catastrophic Health Insurance Act and Medical Assistance Reform Act	1% payroll tax	Covers expenses over $2000	No	No	No
Comprehensive Health Insurance Plan	Employer–employee tax	—	Yes	Share	No
Comprehensive Health Insurance Act	Employer tax; employee voluntary; federal subsidy for poor	—	Yes	Yes; with federal certification of provisions	No
National Health Care Services Reorganization and Reform Act	"	—	Yes	"	No
National Health Care Act	"	—	Yes	"	No
Health Security Act	3.5% payroll tax	—	Yes	None	Yes; amounts appropriated annually

as one of three types: catastrophic insurance for every citizen; comprehensive coverage through private insurance carriers with Federal premium subsidies for the poor; and public compulsory comprehensive insurance. Table 14-1 compares the various proposed bills or plans that have been put forward. A comparison of shifts in support for health care between 1966 and 1975 shows that federal funding is decreasing. Thus, on this basis alone, one is not surprised that numerous plans have been proposed.

Source	1966	1975
State/local	13%	14%
Federal	13	28
Private	74	58

Given that circumstances do affect the priorities for consideration of major proposals by the President and the Congress, National Health Insurance is expected to be among those debated in 1978, if not in connection with bills introduced, most certainly in public forums across the nation, continuing the pattern to date. Some major points of the debate are: whether or not NHI should be compulsory; what the financial base should be; the amount and coverage to be provided; cost-containment measures to be included; and how private citizens may be involved. Most people believe that NHI is inevitable, and recognize that changes in the health care delivery system will develop as a consequence.

Table 14-2 Comparison of Catastrophic and Comprehensive Health Care Plans

Characteristics	Catastrophic	Comprehensive
Coverage	limited	unlimited
Cost	relatively low	high
Access	not affected	increased
Risk to patient	reduced	subsidized
Preventive measures	no incentive for use	use encouraged
Primary care	reduced	increased
Secondary care	increased	reduced

HEALTH PERSONNEL EDUCATION FUNDING

As one of the scarce resources, health personnel has long been the focus of federal efforts to expand the work force and to influence its geographic and social distribution. While dollars are only part of the picture, a review of the levels of federal funding is informative. In 1977–78, the total amount appropriated by a continuing resolution (i.e., maintaining existing authorized programs) was $525 million. The distribution of these funds (in millions of dollars) follows.

Health Professions			Allied Health	
Capitation grants	$144		Special projects	$16.5
Student loans	20		Advanced traineeship	3
Construction	5		Special Projects	
Construction interest			Family medicine, general	
subsidies	2		dentistry	$45
Education loan			Area health education	
repayments	1.5		centers	17
Nursing			Primary care	15
Capitation grants	$ 30		Disadvantaged assistance	14.5
Loans	22.5		MD-Dentist extenders	14
Special projects	15		Emergency med. service	
Nurse practitioner	13		training	6
Traineeships	13		Interdisciplinary training	3.5
Advanced traineeship	12		Financial distress	3
Scholarships	9		Foreign medical student	
Research grants	5		transfers	2
Construction	3.5		Start-up grants	2
Fellowships	1		National Health Service Corps	
Education loan			Scholarship program	$60
repayments	1.5			
Public Health				
Traineeships	$ 7			
Special projects	5			
Health Adm.				
graduate programs	3			
Health Adm. gradu-				
ate traineeships	1.5			

Evidence that federal influence is felt throughout the sphere of health professions education is clearly demonstrated by this listing. Eligibility for federal funds is influenced by many of the legislative provisions for civil rights, regulations governing fiscal accountability, and U.S. Office of Education criteria for recognition of accrediting agencies, to cite a few examples.

As health care continues its progress toward becoming a social service rather than a private commodity, trends for future development indicate that economic support will come primarily from social services rather than the individual. Better organization will be needed in order to make maximal use and distribution of scarce resources.

REFERENCES

1 Anderson, O. and P. Sheatsley, "Comprehensive Medical Insurance," Health Information Foundation Research Series no. 9, New York, 1959.
2 Banks, Peter J., What Canada Has Learned about National Health Insurance, *Prism,* **2:**42–46, January 1974.
3 Davis, K., "National Health Insurance: Benefits, Costs, and Consequences," The Brookings Institution, Washington, D.C., 1975.
4 Mitchell, B. and W. Schwartz, Strategies for Financing National Health Insurance, *N. Eng. J. Med.,* **295:**866–871, Oct. 14, 1976.
5 "National Health Insurance Resource Book," U.S. Government Printing Office, Washington, D.C., 1976.
6 Reinhardt, U., Proposed Changes in the Organization of Health Care Delivery: An Overview and Critique, *Milbank Memorial Fund Quarterly,* Health and Society, **51:**169–222, Fall 1973.
7 Rosett, R. (ed.), "The Role of Health Insurance in Health Services," National Bureau of Economic Research, New York, 1976.
8 "Socioeconomic Issues of Health," Center for Health Services Research and Development, American Medical Association, Chicago, 1977.

Appendix 1

AMERICAN HEART ASSOCIATION
840 North Lake Shore Drive
Chicago, Illinois 60611

STATEMENT ON A PATIENT'S BILL OF RIGHTS
Affirmed by the Board of Trustees November 17, 1972

The American Hospital Association presents a Patient's Bill of Rights with the expectation that observance of these rights will contribute to more effective patient care and greater satisfaction for the patient, his physician, and the hospital organization. Further, the Association presents these rights in the expectation that they will be supported by the hospital on behalf of its patients, as an integral part of the healing process. It is recognized that a personal relationship between the physician and the patient is essential for the provision of proper medical care. The traditional physician-patient relationship takes on a new dimension when care is rendered within an organizational structure. Legal precedent has established that the institution itself also has a responsibility to the patient. It is in recognition of these factors that these rights are affirmed.

1 The patient has the right to considerate and respectful care.

2 The patient has the right to obtain from his physician complete current information concerning his diagnosis, treatment, and prognosis in terms the patient can be reasonably expected to understand. When it is not medically advisable to give such information to the patient, the information should be made available to an appropriate person in his behalf. He has the right to know by name, the physician responsible for coordinating his care.

3 The patient has the right to receive from his physician information necessary to give informed consent prior to the start of any procedure and/or treatment. Except in emergencies, such information for informed consent, should include but not necessarily be limited to the specific procedure and/or treatment, the medically significant risks involved, and the probable duration of incapacitation. Where medically significant alternatives for care or treatment exist, or when the patient requests information concerning medical alternatives, the patient has the right to such information. The patient also has the right to know the name of the person responsible for the procedures and/or treatment.

4 The patient has the right to refuse treatment to the extent permitted by law, and to be informed of the medical consequences of his action.

5 The patient has the right to every consideration of his privacy concerning his own medical care program. Case discussion, consultation, examination, and treatment are confidential and should be conducted discreetly. Those not directly involved in his care must have the permission of the patient to be present.

6 The patient has the right to expect that all communications and records pertaining to his care should be treated as confidential.

7 The patient has the right to expect that within its capacity a hospital must make reasonable response to the request of a patient for services. The hospital must provide evaluation, service, and/or referral as indicated by the urgency of the case. When medically permissible a patient may be transferred to another facility only after he has received complete information and explanation concerning the needs for and alternatives to such a transfer. The institution to which the patient is to be transferred must first have accepted the patient for transfer.

8 The patient has the right to obtain information as to any relationship of his hospital to other health care and educational institutions insofar as his care is concerned. The patient has the right to obtain information as to the existence of any professional relationships among individuals, by name, who are treating him.

9 The patient has the right to be advised if the hospital proposes to engage in or perform human experimentation affecting his care or treatment. The patient has the right to refuse to participate in such research projects.

10   The patient has the right to expect reasonable continuity of care. He has the right to know in advance what appointment times and physicians are available and where. The patient has the right to expect that the hospital will provide a mechanism whereby he is informed by his physician or a delegate of the physician of the patient's continuing health care requirements following discharge.

11   The patient has the right to examine and receive an explanation of his bill regardless of source of payment.

12   The patient has the right to know what hospital rules and regulations apply to his conduct as a patient.

No catalogue of rights can guarantee for the patient the kind of treatment he has a right to expect. A hospital has many functions to perform, including the prevention and treatment of disease, the education of both health professionals and patients, and the conduct of clinical research. All these activities must be conducted with an overriding concern for the patient, and, above all, the recognition of his dignity as a human being. Success in achieving this recognition assures success in the defense of the rights of the patient.

Appendix 2

Health Care and Professional Organizations

Academy of Health Care Consultants
1340 Astor St., Chicago, IL 60610

Ambulance Association of American
Box 11009, Phoenix, AZ 85601

American Academy of Medical Administrators
6 Beacon St., Boston, MA 02108

American Association for Health, Physical
Education and Recreation
1201 16th St. NW, Washington, DC 20036

American Association for Hospital Planning
2284 Main St., Concord, MA 01742

American Association for Laboratory Animal Science
2317 W. Jefferson St., Joliet, IL 60435

American Association for Pastoral Counselors
31 W. 10th St., New York, NY 10011

American Association for Respiratory Therapy
7411 Hines Pl., Dallas, TX 75235

American Association of Blood Banks
1828 L St. NW, Washington, DC 20036

American Association of Certified Orthoptists
Medical University of S. Carolina
80 Barre St., Charleston, SC 29401

American Association of Clinical Chemists
1725 K St. NW, Washington, DC 20006

American Association of Homes for the Aging
374 National Press Bldg. 14th & F Sts.
Washington, DC 20004

American Association of Industrial Nurses, Inc.
79 Madison Ave., New York, NY 10016

American Association of Medical Assistants
1 E. Wacker Dr., Chicago, IL 60601

American Association of Nurse Anesthetists
111 E. Wacker Dr., Chicago, IL 60601

American Association of Volunteer Services Coordinators
18 S. Michigan Ave., Chicago, IL 60603

American Cancer Society
219 E. 42nd St., New York, NY 10017
(see also local chapters)

American Congress of Rehabilitation Medicine
30 N. Michigan Ave., Chicago, IL 60602

American Dental Association
211 E. Chicago Ave., Chicago, IL 60611

American Diabetes Association, Inc.
1 W. 48th St., New York, NY 10020

American Dietetic Association
430 N. Michigan Ave., Chicago, IL 60611

American Electroencephalographic Society
4137 Erie St., Willoughby, OH 44094

American Epilepsy Society
Box 341, Univ. Minn., Minneapolis, MN 55455

American Foundation for the Blind, Inc.
15 W. 16th St., New York, NY 10011

American Health Care Association
1200 15th St. NW, Washington, DC 20005

American Health Foundation
1370 Avenue of the Americas, New York, NY 10019

American Heart Association, Inc.
44 E. 23rd St., New York, NY 10010

American Hospital Association
840 N. Lakeshore Dr., Chicago, IL 60611

American Lung Association
1740 Broadway, New York, NY 10019

American Medical Association
535 N. Dearborn, Chicago, IL 60611

American Medical Record Association
875 N. Michigan, Chicago, IL 60611

American Medical Technologists
710 Higgins Rd., Park Ridge, IL 60068

American National Red Cross
17th & D Sts., Washington, DC 20006

American Nurses' Association
2420 Pershing Rd., Kansas City, MO 64138

American Occupational Therapy Association
6000 Executive Bldg., Rockville, MD 20852

American Osteopathic Association
212 E. Ohio St., Chicago, IL 60611

American Pharmaceutical Association
2215 Constitution Ave., NW, Washington, DC 20037

American Physical Therapy Association
1156 15th St. NW, Washington, DC 20005

American Podiatry Association
20 Chevy Chase Circle NW, Washington, DC 20015

American Psychiatric Association
1700 18th St. NW, Washington, DC 20009

American Psychological Association
1200 17th St. NW, Washington, DC 20036

American Public Health Association, Inc.
1015 18th St. NW, Washington, DC 20037

American Society for Medical Technology
5555 West Loop South, Bellaire, TX 77401

American Society for Microbiology
1913 I St. NW, Washington, DC 20006

American Society of Allied Health Professions
One DuPont Circle, Washington, DC 20036

American Society of Clinical Pathologists
2100 W. Harrison St., Chicago, IL 60612

American Society of Electroencephalographic Technologists
9500 Euclid Ave., Cleveland, OH 44106

American Society of Radiologic Technologists
500 N. Michigan, Chicago, IL 60611

American Speech and Hearing Association
9030 Old Georgetown Rd., Washington, DC 20014

American Veterinary Medicine Association
Mayo Clinic, Rochester, MN 55901

Arthritis Foundation
1212 Avenue of the Americas, New York, NY 10036

Association of Medical Illustrators
6650 Northwest Highway, Chicago, IL 60631

Association of Operating Room Technicians
1100 W. Littleton, Littleton, CO 80120

Biological Photographic Association, Inc.
Box 1057, Rochester, MN 55901

Canadian Arthritis and Rheumatism Society
45 Charles St. E., Toronto, Ont. M4Y 153

Canadian Association of Medical Record Librarians
187 King St. E., Oshawa, Ont. L1H1C3

Canadian Association of Occupational Therapists
4 New Street, Toronto, Ont. M5R 1P6

Canadian Association of Social Workers
55 Parkdale Ave., Ottawa, Ont. K1Y 1E5

Canadian Cancer Society
25 Adelaide St., E. Toronto, 5 Ont.

Canadian Dental Association
234 St. George St., Toronto, Ont. M5R 2P2

Canadian Dietetic Association
1393 Yonge St., Toronto, Ont. M4T 1Y4

Canadian Hearing Society
60 Bedford Rd., Toronto, Ont. M4T 1Y4

Canadian Hospital Association
25 Imperial St., Toronto, Ont. M5P 1C1

Canadian Mental Health Association
2160 Yonge St., Toronto, Ont. M4S 2Z3

Canadian Nurses' Association
CNA House, 50 The Driveway, Ottawa, Ont. K2P 1E2

Canadian Pharmaceutical Association
175 College St., Toronto, Ont. M5T 1P8

Canadian Physiotherapy Association
25 Imperial St., Toronto, Ont. M5P 1B9

Canadian Red Cross Society
95 Wellesly St., E. Toronto, Ont. M4Y 1H6

Canadian Society of Laboratory Technologists
Box 830, Hamilton, Ont. L8N 3N8

Canadian Society of Radiological Technicians
280 Metcalfe St., Ottawa, Ont. K2P 1R7

Group Health Association of America
1717 Massachusetts Ave. NW, Washington, DC 20036

Health Industries Association
111 E. Wacker Dr., Chicago, IL 60606

Health Insurance Association of America
750 Third Ave., New York, NY 10017

Health Law Center,
11600 Nebel St., Rockville, MD 20852

Joint Commission on Accreditation of Hospitals
875 N. Michigan, Chicago, IL 60611

Medical Council of Canada
1867 Alta Vista Dr., Ottawa, Ont. K1G 3H7

Medical Library Association
919 N. Michigan, Chicago, IL 60611

Mental Health Institute
1200 E. Washington, Mt. Pleasant, IA 52641

Muscular Dystrophy Associations of America
810 Seventh Ave., New York, NY 10019

National Ambulance & Medical Services Association
422 Washington Bldg., Washington, DC 20005

National Assembly of National Voluntary Health
Social Welfare Organizations, Inc.
345 E. 46th St., New York, NY 10017

National Association for Hearing and Speech Action
814 Thayer Ave., Silver Spring, MD 20910

National Association for Hospital Development
Box 829, Topeka, KS 66601

National Association for Mental Health, Inc.
1800 N. Kent St., Arlington, VA 22209

National Association for Music Therapy
Box 610, Lawrence, KS 66044

National Association for Retarded Citizens
2709 Avenue E East, Arlington, TX 76011

National Association of Home Health Agencies
605 Bannock St., Denver, CO 80204

National Association of Patients on Hemodialysis
and Transplants
505 Northern Blvd., Great Neck, NY 11201

National Association of Sheltered Workshops and
Homebound Programs
5530 Wisconsin Ave., Washington, DC 22015

National Association of Social Workers, Inc.
600 Southern Blvd., 15th & H Sts., Washington, DC 20005

National Center for Voluntary Action
1785 Massachusetts Ave. NW, Washington, DC 20036

National Council for International Health
Box 4909, Chicago, IL 60680

National Council on Alcoholism, Inc.
2 Park Ave., New York, NY 10016

National Council on the Aging,
1828 L St. NW, Washington, DC 20036

National Easter Seal Society for Crippled Children and Adults
2023 W. Ogden Ave., Chicago, IL 60612

National Environmental Health Association
1600 Pennsylvania Ave., Denver, CO 80203

National Foundation
1275 Mamaroneck Ave., White Plains, NY 10605

National Health Council, Inc.
1740 Broadway, New York, NY 10019

National Hemophilia Foundation
1740 Broadway, New York, NY 10019

National Kidney Foundation
116 E. 27th St., New York, NY 10016

National Medical Association, Inc.
2109 E St. NW, Washington, DC 20037

National Multiple Sclerosis Society
257 Park Ave., New York, NY 10010

National Parkinson Foundation, Inc.
1501 NW Ninth Ave., Miami, FL 33136

National Society for Prevention of Blindness
79 Madison Ave., New York, NY 10016

United Cerebral Palsy Associations, Inc.
66 E. 34th St., New York, NY 10016

World Health Organization
Regional Office for the Americas
525 23rd St. NW, Washington, DC 20037

INDEX

Page numbers in *italic* indicate tables.